WE'VE LOST MY PROSTATE, MATE!
And life goes on ...

Alan White

First published by Busybird Publishing 2016
Copyright © 2016 Alan White

ISBN
Print: 978-0-9945839-6-3
Ebook: 978-0-9945839-7-0

Alan White has asserted his right under the Copyright, Designs and Patents Act 1988 to be identified as the author of this work. The information in this book is based on the author's experiences and opinions. The publisher specifically disclaims responsibility for any adverse consequences, which may result from use of the information contained herein. Permission to use information has been sought by the author. Any breaches will be rectified in further editions of the book.

All rights reserved. No part of this publication may be reproduced, stored in or introduced into a retrieval system, or transmitted in any form, or by any means (electronic, mechanical, photocopying, recording or otherwise) without the prior written permission of the author. Any person who does any unauthorised act in relation to this publication may be liable to criminal prosecution and civil claims for damages. Enquiries should be made through the publisher.

Cartoons: Lianne Kernahan
Cover image: Justin Leijon
Cover design: Ai Tsuruma
Layout and typesetting: Busybird Publishing

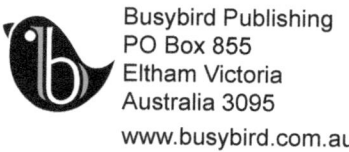

Busybird Publishing
PO Box 855
Eltham Victoria
Australia 3095
www.busybird.com.au

Testimonials

"Alan's candid account of his journey reflects his obvious passion for empowering men. His story is reader friendly, infused with good humour and an enormous sense of empathy. It encapsulates not only the practical aspects of managing the diagnosis but references the variety of conventional and alternative treatments available. Implications for quality of life and especially intimate relationships are also presented with an astounding honesty. This is an enlightening read for any man diagnosed with prostate cancer, their family members and clinicians working in the field."
	Ms Sarah Rudd
	APA Continence and Women's Health Physiotherapist
	Women's and Men's Health Physiotherapy, Hampton

"Alan is such a committed practitioner, so it made perfect sense for him to write this book; in order to benefit men and their families in understanding the process of prostate cancer.

"His informative and somewhat humorous take on his cancer certainly helps reduce the fear factor. Fiona's story is invaluable from a partner's perspective. The silver lining, as well as, Alan's remission would be the strengthening of Alan and Fiona's relationship."
	Cynthia Chenier-Hinde
	Consultant

Loved the book - it's not easy for men to have first-hand information about the diagnosis and treatment of prostate cancer. Your personal account provides some of the emotional impacts not available in a clinical setting.

Roy Francis,
Founder and Secretary/Convenor of the Mornington Peninsula Prostate Cancer Support Group

In this book Alan describes in great detail his journey and experiences with prostate cancer, from his early diagnosis in 2000 followed by active surveillance for 10 years and the ultimate treatment of his cancer through robotic laparoscopic prostatectomy. It's a warts and all story covering his first hand experiences dealing with emotions, social and practical issues of the side effects of erectile dysfunction and incontinence. His experiences are very intimate and detailed and provide an insight on how Alan and his wife Fiona have overcome many problems realising there is light at the end of the tunnel through making life-changing decisions on the way and being capably supported by family and friends. In writing this book Alan has also drawn on resources/books relevant to his journey and experiences. Despite the serious nature of the topic, Alan has maintained a sense of humour as reflected by the cartoons in the various sections of the book.

This book is a valuable resource for any newly diagnosed man considering surgical intervention for his prostate cancer and having to contemplate resulting side effects such as erectile dysfunction and incontinence. The book provides encouragement, hope and ideas for the best outcome and maintenance of quality of life.

Wolfgang Schoch
Prostate Cancer Survivor, PCFA Ambassador and Support Group Leader of Prostate Melbourne, Victoria

Alan and I are friends who met when we both became Ambassador Speakers for the Prostate Cancer Foundation. Both of us have been through prostate cancer procedures and, although my path was different to Alan's, the book brought up lots of similarities in the emotions involved before and after treatment. Alan has always been such a positive person in the time I have known him and he is always completely down to earth. This practical down to earth approach really comes through in this book. Most importantly the book touches on subjects that are not always covered in dealing with cancer – i.e. the emotional aspects which we experience in coming to terms with this illness. I thoroughly recommend this book to anyone who is touched by prostate issues – either themselves or in their loved ones. Well done Alan in writing such an insightful book.
    Rod Smith
    Prostate Cancer Survivor, PCFA Ambassador, Victoria

Well done, Alan and Fiona.

    This is an easy to read, informative and very educational book about a very complex issue. Written in layman's language that explains complicated medical topics extremely well. All men, and their partners, should read this excellent guide book!
    Pete Fraser

Contents

Disclaimer	i
Acknowledgements	iii
Preface	v
1. Understanding the Male Anatomy	1
2. My Diagnosis	5
3. We've Only Just Met!	13
4. The Operation and the Aftermath	19
5. Let the Healing Begin	27
6. Wake-Up Calls, with the Advantage of Hindsight	43
7. Dressing Percy	51
8. The Measuring Cup	59
9. So Many Problems Solved	61
10. What We All Want to Know	65
11. Trial, Error and Success	69
12. Consequences	73
13. Coming to Terms with Change	79
14. A Wife's Perspective – Over to Fiona	87
15. Be Kind to Yourself and Ask for Help	91
16. There is Light at the End of the Tunnel	93
17. Things to Consider If Diagnosed with Prostate Cancer	97
Postscript: Two Years On	103
Postscript: Five Years On	107
Final Word from Fiona – Five Years On	115
References	119
Resources	121

Disclaimer

The contents of this book do not purport to offer any medical advice whatsoever to the reader.

Any man who may be having issues with his bladder, prostate or sexual function, or experiencing any other health concerns, needs to seek advice from a qualified health professional pertaining to his own circumstances.

It is also not the intention of this book to support one form of treatment over another, as there are ongoing advances occurring in the different fields of medicine, and those therapies that are being used to treat prostate cancer here in Australia and overseas.

At the time of publishing, pathologists currently use the Gleason scoring system to grade the level of cancer within the prostate. The Royal College of Pathology in Australia and New Zealand has recently accepted a new standard of grading. The World Health Organisation (WHO) has also accepted the revised scoring system. The original Gleason score will continue to be used alongside the new grading system. Where the Gleason score is mentioned in this book, it refers to the older system that was in place at the time of my diagnosis.

Each man needs to discuss the options and possible outcomes with his specialist(s); and this discussion will be influenced by what stage the prostate cancer is at for each individual.

This is a story of my own journey and experiences, as well as information that I have gleaned along the way, some of which has come from talking to other men when doing presentations on men's health, who have also been dealing with prostate related issues that affected them physically, emotionally, and within their relationships.

I have also included the practicalities of dealing with the day-to-day recovery and what I found worked for me. Along the way, I have come across men and their partners who have demonstrated courage, humour, honesty, vulnerability, and a willingness to talk and share their experiences with others. Having a sense of humour when dealing with prostate cancer, from my point of view, helps one to get through each day – not that it's a laughing matter, losing your prostate, mate!

Acknowledgements

There have been many people who have been very supportive over the years, from when I was initially diagnosed with suspected prostate cancer back in 1996 while living in Albury-Wodonga, such as Elsie and Michael Pobjoy, members of the local Reiki group, Ginny and Michael Bydder and many others.

Then, in 2000, I had returned to Melbourne to live, when having a check-up on my prostate I was diagnosed with prostate cancer with a PSA of 10 and a Gleason score of 6. I am thankful for the support from my partner at the time, Joy, and the staff at the Hilton on The Park Spa complex, where I was working.

In 2011, when the prostate cancer decided to return, following ten years of active surveillance, I had to make a hard decision. There were my family; staunch friends Robert and Cynthia Hinde, Peter Fraser, Doug and Kate Parkinson, Kaylene and Brian Andrews, Charlie Brown, Stan and Dianne Harris; committee members of the Royal Australian Air Force Vietnam Veterans' Association; board members of the Air Force Association (Vic); along with Professor Tony Costello, his nurse Helen Crowe, and my GP, Dr Robyn Green, all in support.

After the operation, I had the help of The Women's and Men's Health Physiotherapy Group, in particular Rebecca and Sarah; Dr Eric Dowker, Chiropractor; Kate Madigan, Reflexologist; Dr David Wang, Acupuncturist; as well as Dr Kristen Manallack and Dr Eliza Gleadell, Osteopaths.

Our friend Lianne Kernahan made a special contribution to this book, in the form of her cartoons, provided along with her sense of humour, patience and suggestions whenever I wanted her to make changes to the drawings.

No book would be complete without an engaging cover. My thanks go to our friend, Ai Tsuruma, of Pudding Creative, for her excellent designs and creative input. I also want to thank Ai's partner, Justin Leijon, for his outstanding photography and ability to make us look good.

Finally I would to like to offer a big, deeply heart-felt thank you to my wife, Fiona, for her unfailing love, support, encouragement, sense of humour, and willingness to remain intimate. I am also grateful for her skill and input to this book by way of layout, editing and suggestions. Fiona did whatever was necessary, physically and emotionally, so that I would not feel I was any less a man, just because I was unable to gain an erection, and dealing with incontinence in the months following the operation. My enduring love for you always.

Preface

This story had been in the back of my mind for a couple of years or more, instigated by my own experience of prostate cancer and of conducting active surveillance for ten years prior to the operation. It is a bit of a warts and all story concerning my experiences in the months that followed the operation. Hopefully some of this information will prepare the reader in some way, should they, in the future, face a similar experience.

I was influenced also by my involvement for over ten years with the Department of Veterans' Affairs (DVA) as a Men's Health Peer Educator (MHPE), presenting information to ex-service organisations on health and wellbeing and talking to men about their health, especially prostate issues.

I have also been involved for over four years with the Prostate Cancer Foundation Australia (PCFA) as a Men's Health Ambassador Speaker, delivering presentations on prostate health and wellbeing to a wide variety of public and private organisations. Delivering talks to these organisations gave me the privilege of talking to individual men who, having had the prostate operation, felt they just needed to talk things over, and maybe these talks provided them with their first opportunity to do so.

And, of course, there was *Movember*, for the previous three years, with a team of fellow Bros, growing the Mo to raise funds, increase public awareness around prostate cancer, and to encourage men to take care of their health and wellbeing.

Then there is the local Bayside Kingston Prostate Cancer Support Group, where I was further privileged to meet men who had their own experiences and treatments; the good, the bad and the ugly.

All these connections and experiences were bubbling away in my mind, but I was not really sure what exactly I would have to say or contribute to men's understanding about prostate cancer.

For every man who is diagnosed with prostate cancer, each will have a different prognosis. A man's treatment will be influenced accordingly by his age, genetic background, general health, and whatever stage the cancer has reached. The level of the Prostate Specific Antigen (PSA) that is present in his blood sample will also be a factor, along with anything that the digital rectal examination reveals, as well as the results from any biopsy of the prostate. All these matters will need to be considered in relation to treatment.

So, it is a matter of having the right attitude and mind-set towards your own health and wellbeing, not just for your own sake, but for your family too. There is also the ripple effect that comes from having been diagnosed with prostate cancer that affects your partner and family.

As I have always stated at the many talks I have given over the years, make visiting your doctor a normal part of your life. Develop a relationship with him/her, get your figures done regularly; this means your blood pressure, cholesterol levels, glucose levels (diabetes), plus your weight/waist measurement. If you have a family history of prostate disease, it is my opinion that you should have your PSA levels (and free-to-total PSA) checked once you reach the age of 40. This will give you a baseline from which you can monitor your PSA levels. If you have no family history of prostate disease, it is generally considered that 50 years of age is the appropriate starting point for annual PSA checks, along with a digital rectal examination to check the condition of the prostate and rectal area.

Taking care of your health and wellbeing includes exercising regularly and observing your food intake – energy in, energy out – as this affects your weight. You also need to watch your alcohol intake and stop smoking. Reduce your saturated fat intake, make sure you eat plenty of fruit and vegetables, complex carbohydrates – i.e. not processed stuff – and lean protein.

It is important to have a varied diet and, of course, drink plenty of water to keep hydrated. And most importantly, keep your stress levels to a minimum, as constant and chronic stress will impact on your immune system's ability to deal with any infections and inflammation that arise in your body.

Getting your figures done establishes a baseline from which you can see how you are tracking with your health each year. Then you, and your doctor, can pick up any early changes in any of those figures, and take appropriate action. Make sure that you get a copy of the results so you have a record also.

1. Understanding the Male Anatomy

A number of men are probably not fully conversant with what the prostate does, or any of the other parts that make up the male reproductive system. So here is a brief overview; all male mammals have a prostate. Interestingly, it seems only men and male dogs have a problem with the prostate. I wonder what that means?

The prostate gland is about the size and shape of a walnut. It is attached to the underneath of the bladder, whilst surrounding the urethra which is attached to the bladder, deep within the pelvic region. The prostate provides nutrition for the sperm, along with secretions that make up the ejaculation fluid. The seminal vesicles located on top of the prostate also provide secretions to this fluid.

The testicles (your balls) produce testosterone – the male hormone – and in the epididymis the sperm – those little tadpole-looking wrigglers – are produced. When you are about to ejaculate, the sperm travel up the vas deferens, with fluid being added to them by the seminal vesicles and the prostate. Then they travel out via the ejaculatory duct down into the urethra and out through the penis.

Urine from the bladder is drained by the urethra through the prostate and, as men age, some may experience the prostate becoming enlarged and squeezing the urethra, thus interfering with the flow of urine through the prostate. There is medication and surgery that can deal with this problem. Symptoms include stop-start flow of urine, frequent urination, dribbling or having to get up throughout the night to visit the toilet. There can be a variety of reasons for these symptoms, so go to the doctor for an examination as this sort of thing does not go away, but it does not necessarily mean you have cancer!

A problem facing men after surgery or radiation therapy is that of incontinence. With radiation it's generally due to the burning effect of the treatment, but with surgery it's more to do with what is removed with the urethra within the prostate, and that is the internal urethral sphincter.

The term *urethral sphincter* refers to one of two muscles used to control the exit of urine in the urinary bladder through the urethra. The two muscles are the external urethral sphincter and the internal urethral sphincter. When either of these muscles contract, the urethra is sealed shut.

When the prostate is removed, so is the internal urethral sphincter, and along with that goes the involuntary or automatic control of the flow of urine.

The external urethral sphincter is the one that men have to control via exercises for the pelvic floor muscle to strengthen the area and the sphincter muscle. During surgery there may be some damage to the pudendal nerve which is involved in urine control and this can take some time to heal.

In males, the internal sphincter muscle of the urethra functions to prevent backflow of seminal fluids into the bladder during ejaculation. Some men may find that they experience this backflow after a re-bore of the urethra.

During surgery to remove the prostate, the surgeon will either cut or clip the vas deferens so that there will no longer be any seminal fluid (including sperm) travelling from the testicles during orgasm. In other words, you can still have an orgasm but you will not be ejaculating any fluid sperm.

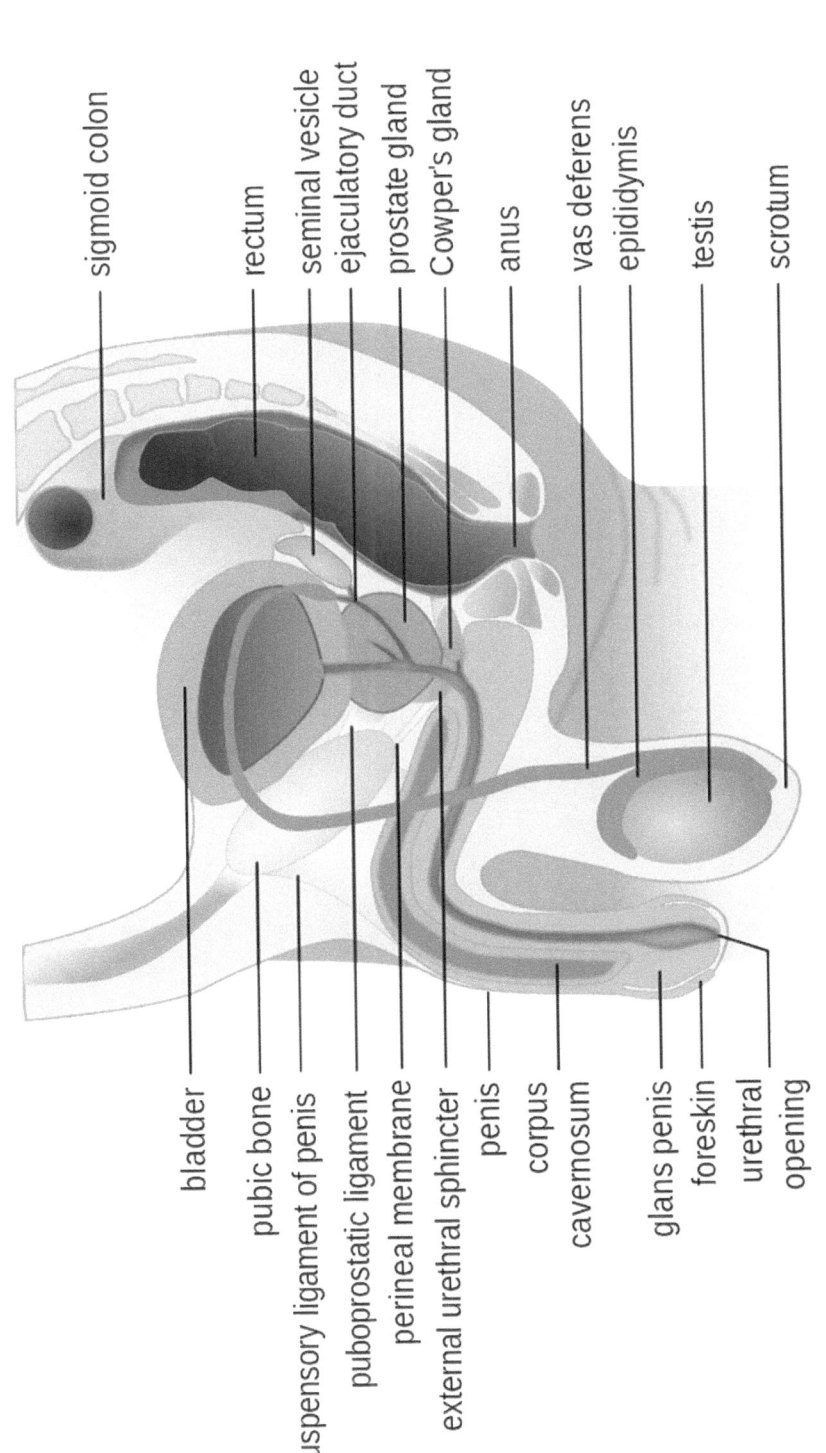

2. My Diagnosis

In November 2010, I had my regular blood test to check my Prostate Specific Antigen (PSA) level, and the other usual figures. A week later the results came back and the score/level was 1.9, which for my age – 60 years at the time – was not high. Interestingly, between 2008 and up to 2011, my PSA had been up and down, going from 1.8 in 2007, to 1.1 in 2008, to 1.4 mid 2009, and in 2010 it was 1.5.

So, in November 2010, when those results came back showing 1.9, I got a sense that something wasn't right, despite the GP saying that no action was required. Again, the level was not high; I had been doing active surveillance for the previous ten years, and the PSA had been fairly low during that period.

Active surveillance is an alternative to current medical treatments that not all men know about. It is an approach that is becoming more widespread for men who meet specific criteria. Generally speaking, men whose biopsy results show a localised, low-grade, low-risk prostate cancer can look at this option. Active surveillance avoids the immediate side-effects from treatment, such as incontinence, infertility and erectile dysfunction. It is always best for men to discuss all possible treatment options, including active surveillance, with their specialist physician.

Now, on reflection, I realise that I had been getting cold sores regularly and had been stressed out for a number of years, although I felt I was staying on top most of the time, and taking the appropriate supplements. Yet something was not right; had the immune system been under too much stress for too long? Yes, I was 60, and the PSA for my age can creep up, but why? There was a nagging doubt at the back of my mind about what was going on.

In the following month, December 2010, I had my regular visit to see my urologist, Professor Tony Costello, which included a digital rectal examination, or *DRE*. As it had been a few years since I had a biopsy of the prostate, Tony decided to do one in January 2011. This time there would be an anaesthetic so I would be out to it; thank goodness for that!

This procedure went well. I was a bit sore for a day or so after, but it certainly was easier than having a biopsy while being awake. My wife, Fiona, and I met with Tony a week later to get the results from the biopsy. Helen, his nurse, was also in the room when Tony came in. For an instant I thought that was a bit strange, but then Tony said he had the results – the cancer was back!

I looked at Fiona and then back at Tony. I was glad she was with me. I said that was not what I was expecting. Tony stated that he was not surprised, as the gland had felt firm when he did the DRE back in December. Funnily enough, I did not ask how the prostate felt at the time of the DRE, and Tony didn't comment either, which was odd. We discussed the Gleason scores of the core samples from the prostate biopsy. These cores had multi-focal scores of 6 (being 3 + 3) and a score of 7 which was deemed to be aggressive. The PSA had been only 1.9 – thank goodness I had a biopsy. Now I was between a rock and a hard place, with active surveillance no longer an option due to the prostate showing aggressive cells.

The *Gleason score* refers to a grading system used by the pathologist when they examine tissue taken from the prostate to determine how aggressive the cancer is likely to be. The PSA and the Gleason score may not always match; in that you can have a low PSA (say, 3-4) and a Gleason score of around 6-7; or it can be any combination. The Gleason score is discussed in more detail later on in this book. In 2011, my free-to-total score for PSA was running around 12%; anything below 25% may indicate the possibility of cancer in the prostate. I clearly had not been checking my free-to-total PSA levels regularly.

So, even with a low PSA, there may be other factors to consider, such as whether the prostate feels firm or lumpy. PSA is a protein which is secreted by the cells in the gland of the prostate, and a high reading can be due to any number of reasons and does not always mean that there is prostate cancer present. It may mean there is an infection, or you may have an enlarged prostate that is pumping out more PSA than usual. It's useful to have a second test done somewhere between three and six weeks later to check the level again.

Part of me had thought, during the week following the biopsy, well if the cancer does come back it will be small, and I will do what I did before to deal with the cancer. This time, however, I am not so sure.

Tony wanted to start things rolling. I needed time to get my head around what had happened and why – what was different this time? Had I been slack in looking after my health? Had there been too much ongoing stress for the last, well, ten years and, in particular, the last couple of years? Now, on reflection, I feel that this may well have played a part, as ongoing stress will impact on the immune system.

I wanted to look at options, and as I was talking to Helen, Tony's urology nurse, about what papers I needed to fill in, it felt like everything was moving way too quickly. Helen suggested that I see an incontinence physiotherapist for specific exercises pre- and post-operation. The suggested physiotherapy practice was close to home so I didn't have to go far.

Every time I reflect on that day, I am still not sure what I was feeling. A bit numb? Confused and blank? I think I was a bit separated from my body for a while, and went into autopilot, with my left brain attempting to work out what to do next. Getting the prostate out was not my desired option, yet. Tony stuck his head around the door and said, with a grin, something to the effect, "Don't let him out without the papers signed".

The next two weeks or so were a bit surreal. I had an appointment with the physiotherapist to check me out. I was attempting to look at other options, and did not feel particularly strong about having another go at alternative methods to deal with prostate cancer this time round. Now, when I reflect on that time, I realise that active surveillance or taking the alternative therapy route were no longer viable options. With aggressive cells sitting within the prostate, I could not possibly know how long it would be before they could spread and go walk-about.

Being diagnosed with prostate cancer, I felt at times as if I was walking around inside a bubble, separate from everyone and from day-to-day events. Sometimes, I would walk down the street feeling that I wanted to yell at people – "I've been diagnosed with prostate cancer!" I wanted people to acknowledge somehow that a major change was occurring in my life.

Then there was the decision regarding who to tell about the results and the treatment to be undertaken. Two days after meeting Tony and being confronted by the return of the cancer, I had to take my mother to a skin specialist to have some stitches removed, as she had had an operation on her leg to remove a couple of skin cancers the week before. As I was driving her to the appointment, she asked what the result of my visit to the urologist was. I was not ready to tell her at that point, and was thinking that she might have forgotten and would be preoccupied with her own health concerns.

As I was a bit caught out and didn't think quickly enough to delay my answer, I told her and she was upset – understandably so. Over the years, my mum had her own ongoing skin cancer problems, and was tiring of the treatments that she had been having.

I was not in a good space to be dealing with mum's

2. My Diagnosis

emotions as well; however, having to support her while the stitches were removed, rather reluctantly, this took my mind off my own stuff and focused me on supporting mum and getting her through the procedure that day. Once that was over though, how does one go about telling other family, friends? I didn't want them finding out after the event, but was not looking for sympathy either.

So, as I made the calls to let others know what was going on, I had this strange feeling as if I was ringing people up to let them know I had won TattsLotto! Now that was weird. I was only ringing family and close friends whom I had known for some time, but all the same it did feel rather surreal to be calling people up to say, "Hey, guess what? My prostate cancer is back, and it's coming out, so now I will have lost my cherry twice!"

In Vietnam, the local women who worked in the Vung Tau Air Force Base would say to the new arrivals, "You are a cherry boy." This was because the lads hadn't yet been into town to lose their virginity. The local women seemed to know who had and who hadn't been into town (Vung Tau). Thus my reference to losing my cherry twice – I referred to my prostate as the cherry – you've got to have some humour around the situation.

Of course, everybody was surprised, as I was, but I remained upbeat about my decision and outcomes, for their sake as well as mine. With some of the friends I rang, we talked about what I had done previously in dealing with the earlier prostate cancer, and whether I would be taking the approach of active surveillance again. This time I knew that I could not avoid having my prostate removed. It just remained for me to decide on the path – surgery or radiation therapy.

During the period leading up to the operation, I remember walking on the beach one morning, reviewing the events leading up to where I was then, not knowing what to do and crying at what I thought was the unfairness of what I was experiencing after all those years of surveillance.

Yet, in the months following the operation, I would often question myself as to whether it was the right decision; this was something I had to stop doing as it was not helpful or conducive to my healing on different levels. Even in mid-2011, when I finally did get to see Dr Eric Dowker (chiropractor), to work on the problems I was having, I thought then, "Why didn't I come to see Eric sooner, like before the operation, or even sooner after the operation?" Again, it was not very helpful to dwell on the past.

I decided to look at options, with one of them being *Brachytherapy*. This procedure involves the placement of radioactive pellets/seeds within the prostate gland. There are two major forms of Brachytherapy; one involves a permanent, low-dose-rate seed insertion into the prostate, and the other method is a temporary high-dose-rate into the prostate.

Generally speaking, a man who is diagnosed with localised, low risk prostate cancer may be eligible for this type of treatment. From my reading, most literature cites the eligibility criteria as being: a PSA of less than 10, Gleason score below 8, a life expectancy of greater than 10 years, a prostate size of 20-50mls, and minimal urinary symptoms.

For further information on this, I recommend the book *Prostate Cancer, Your guide to the disease, treatment options and outcomes*, by Associate Professor Prem Rashid, 3rd edition. This book is very worthwhile for a review of all treatments and a good source of information for men about the prostate in general; even if you don't have any problems, it's useful as a resource guide.

Another useful guide is the newsletter put out by the Prostate Cancer Foundation Australia (PCFA), which reviews current treatments, their outcomes and new innovations that are being developed in the treatment of prostate cancer, here in Australia and overseas.

I also looked at the after-effects of Brachytherapy and, from my reading; some men do eventually end up with incontinence issues and erectile dysfunction due to the nerves eventually being cooked by the radiation seeds. That means some men will need to inject into their penis to gain an erection, or take Viagra™, or use a vacuum device. Again,

2. My Diagnosis

every man is different and will respond to each treatment differently.

I had another meeting with Tony to discuss the options and, after some serious conversation, it was decided that Robotic Radical Prostatectomy surgery would be the treatment for me. As my Gleason score showed aggressive cells, my situation could not be described as "low risk" and was therefore not suitable for radiation therapy. Tony stated that his first concern was to keep me alive and that meant removing the prostate. After the operation, it would be getting the incontinence under control and then dealing with the erection problem. Tony believed that, with the appropriate exercises, the incontinence would be rectified and, within two years, my erections would be up and running!

He also stated that ten years ago I had made the right decision at the time for me, for now I would be getting Robotic surgery, as Tony had pioneered this form of treatment for the last ten years, so he knew what he was doing.

Luckily for me, the Department of Veterans' Affairs (DVA) would cover all expenses as the Department had accepted the prostate cancer as being related to my war service. So, into Helen's office to fill in the paperwork, and then Tony stuck his head through the door to say, "Tie his leg to the chair this time, so he doesn't leave without the paperwork." As Fiona and I left, we spoke to Tony again, who quipped "I told you I'd get your prostate one day."

I know that this is an expensive operation for men to pay for; however, I am aware that certain public hospitals are attempting to get the Robotic equipment into their operating rooms, not just for prostate surgery, but also for other types of operations.

3. We've Only Just Met!

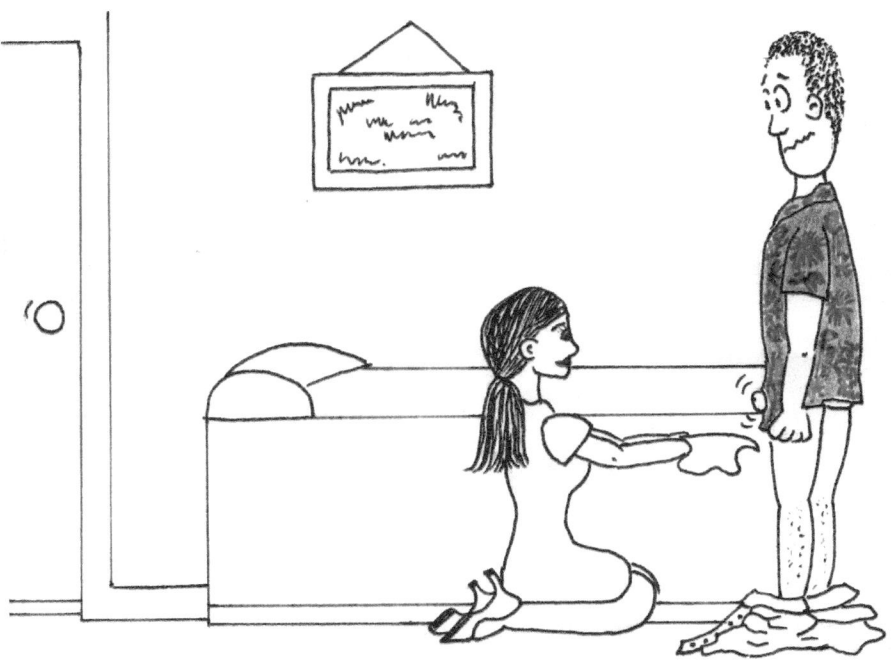

A visit to the physiotherapist was interesting. We discussed my background, previous operations including a re-bore of the bladder, or as it is called a *Trans-Urethral Resection of the Prostate* (TURP). The physiotherapist, Rebecca, explained that she would have to examine the pelvic floor muscle to get an idea of its tone. As she said this, I was thinking there was only one way you can do that!

So I got up on the couch, lowered my jocks, and lay on my side, pulling my knees up to my chest. Rebecca inserted a gloved finger into my rectum, explaining she would not be feeling my prostate; not that I would complain. After having had Tony's large finger do the same procedure, Rebecca's finger was a lot easier to tolerate.

Also, Fiona had come along so that she could understand what would be happening, and she was sitting in the room behind the curtain while Rebecca was examining me. I wondered what she was thinking about with a beautiful young woman sticking her finger up my bum!

As Rebecca felt the area, she discovered that the pelvic floor muscle was too tight, and this probably explained the shooting pain I would get from time to time right up the middle of my rectum. In fact, the pelvic floor felt uncomfortable when she touched it, and there was a trigger point in the area which felt very Ouchy when probed.

Rebecca also checked my lower abdominals to see how effectively I could pull up my pelvic floor muscles. For some time I had been practising a simple pelvic floor movement, which is basically being able to activate them and, in turn, I was then able to raise or pull up Percy to some degree – if the exercise was done properly. This movement should also enable you to stop the urine flow mid-stream.

At another appointment, Rebecca actually had me stand up with my jocks off, and watched me as I activated the pelvic floor to check the movement of my penis. She also had her hand underneath my penis, holding a tissue in case there were any unfortunate dribbles!

I was given specific pelvic floor exercises to do, but I also had to focus on letting go and relaxing the pelvic floor after each exercise. These exercises were to be performed to assist in managing the incontinence which would occur after the operation.

Background on PSA, Gleason and Scores

Having an elevated PSA does not mean that the prostate has cancer, but it is an indicator that there may be a problem with the gland. It may be that the prostate is enlarged and secreting extra PSA protein, or it may be Benign Prostate Enlargement (BPE). The man may have had sex the night before the blood sample is taken, which can stimulate the prostate to produce additional PSA. Remember; do not have sex for at least three days before a blood test for PSA. Levels can go up and down for no reason at all and if you happen to have a large prostate, that in itself may contribute to a possible higher PSA reading.

It is also advisable to have your blood test for PSA **prior to** having a DRE, as the DRE itself can stimulate the gland to produce more PSA.

If your PSA level is elevated, the doctor may then perform a Digital Rectal Examination (DRE). This involves the doctor passing a gloved finger into your rectum (back passage) to feel for any abnormalities in the back passage or on the prostate gland.

Another possible explanation for higher PSA levels is that you may be experiencing prostatitis, which is an inflammatory condition of the prostate that may cause a rise in the PSA.

This would need to be confirmed by your doctor or urologist and, if prostatitis is present, it needs to be treated as the infection will not go away, and you will probably require a treatment of antibiotics.

If you are experiencing ongoing elevated PSA levels, and the prostate gland on examination is felt to be firm or lumpy, then you may be referred to a urologist for further examination and possibly a biopsy of the prostate.

This is generally done under anaesthetic, but not all the time. Samples of tissue are taken from the prostate, and then sent to pathology for examination to determine whether or not they are cancerous. It is from this procedure that the pathologist gives what is called a Gleason score, to determine the level of cancer present in the tissue samples.

> Prostate cancer cells are graded by a numerical scoring system called the Gleason grade which range from 1 to 5 (the lower the grade, the lesser the potential level of aggression) (Rashid, p56). The Gleason score (range 2 to 10) is calculated by adding the two most common grades on the biopsy sample.
>
> Staging is important to help determine the plan of treatment. It is about trying to establish how involved the cancer is within the prostate, and assess its progression, outside the confines of the prostate... The system that is mostly used now is the TNM system. (Rashid, p66)

Most men will hear of grading such as T1 through to T4. As Rashid explains:

> **T1** is when the tumour is small and **cannot be felt** with a finger examination (rectal examination or ultrasound). It is found either during a TURP (prostate rebore surgery) or biopsy... **T2** is when the tumour can be **felt** but is **confined** within the prostate... **T3** is when the tumour extends beyond the prostate capsule and/or is spreading into the adjacent structures called **seminal vesicles**... **T4** is when it is spreading beyond the seminal vesicles and into adjacent organs like the bladder, rectum or pelvis. (Rashid, p66)

At this point, I would like to add that the above is only a guide and that every man will have different findings, and possibly not even fit into the above classifications. I certainly did not fit the average picture, starting with a low PSA of 1.9, and the biopsy I had showed agressive cancer cells.

It is a fact that most men will die in old age from other causes, such as cardiovascular problems, smoking-related issues, skin cancer, or any of a number of diseases, or accidents. Yet their prostate will most likely have traces of cancer within its confines. These men may not be experiencing any of the possible symptoms related to prostate cancer, or even have any problems whatsoever.

Some background might be useful to illustrate how I came to reach this particular stage of my life – losing my prostate gland, and having to deal with incontinence and erectile dysfunction.

4. The Operation and the Aftermath

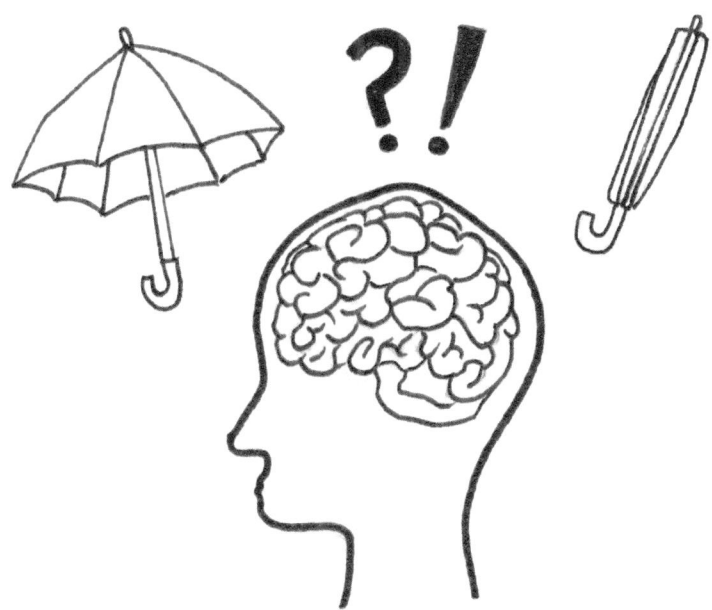

Looking at the above picture, ask yourself what is the connection between the two? If you were in the rain, would the umbrella work if it was closed?

Every day we are challenged to take in new information, change and adapt to what is occurring around for us, at home, work, personally, and in the environment in which we live.

So, would your brain work if it were not open to taking in information?

All I am asking of you, the reader, is to allow your brain to be like the umbrella; be open to what follows and, if you don't agree, then that's fine, just let that particular piece of information go through to the wicketkeeper! You may feel that it's not relevant to you and that's okay too. When you are finished with this book, please pass it on to your mate, father, brother, uncle, nephew, or any clubs you are involved with; help to spread the word wide and far.

Let the Story Unfold!

In the tradition of Australian laconic humour, let me first relate the following incident.

'A funny thing happened on the way to the operating theatre'. It was Tuesday, mid-afternoon on February 8, 2011. The anaesthetist had put a shunt into my upper left arm and given me a sedative, I think. Anyway, as I was being wheeled into the operating room, I had a sudden sense of 'What the fuck was I thinking?'

Then I saw the robot, covered in sterile plastic, looming at the end of the operating table, looking like something out of *Doctor Who*.

It was February, my wife's birthday that month, Valentine's Day, and our wedding anniversary too. Here I was about to be operated on to remove my prostate! Flow-on results would include incontinence and erectile dysfunction (no nookies!). I believe some men do not experience these problems for very long after the operation, yet each of us will respond and heal differently when faced with these two issues.

I related this insight to the anaesthetist, and we both laughed about the timing of the operation, but it was a bit late to be rescheduling. He also commented that I seemed a bit young to be having the operation; I could not agree more; but 'shit happens'. Well, at least we got to celebrate our wedding anniversary, if you get my drift (that means sex).

4. The Operation and the Aftermath

These thoughts and other ideas for this book were cascading through my mind very early (1:40am) on Wednesday morning, 9 February, 2011, while I was laid up in bed at the Epworth Hospital, Richmond. I was recovering from robotic-assisted laparoscopic radical prostatectomy surgery; that is a mouthful. I usually call it robotic prostate removal.

Resting in bed later that morning, I was thinking about going home soon, as my wife, Fiona, and our friend, Kate, were coming to pick me up. Catering staff were doing the rounds with breakfast, but I was not feeling in the mood. Then I started to realise that I felt nauseous. There was a small container/bowl on the bed, but as I leaned forward to sit up and use it, my abdomen did not want to function; this was due to the incisions that had been made through the abdominal muscles.

So, I was leaning to the side and throwing up. A nurse came in and gave me one of those plastic sick bags, and off I went again. The nurse then gave me a shot in the arm to settle down the nausea, and hooked me up to a drip. I was not feeling flash at all.

Not long after, Professor Tony Costello, my urologist, arrived to check in with me. He took one look and said words to the effect, "You don't look too flash".

I told him that I was given a combination of morphine and sedative by the anaesthetist in the lower back just prior to the operation. The reason for the morphine was to help relax the bladder, and reduce any spasm occurring after the operation. Also, taking medication for the spasm orally won't reach the bladder. I remember him saying as he was about to inject me, "There might be a bit of a sting". Being slightly relaxed already, I didn't feel a thing, and then I was out to it.

Tony suggested that I had experienced a reaction to the morphine/sedative; either way, I would not be going home that day, and I started to throw up again. Fiona and Kate arrived mid-morning and, on seeing my state, realised I was not going home with them so off they went to have a coffee without me!

I continued to feel nauseous, and continued to receive a number of injections to reduce the nausea, plus the drip-line was hooked up to my arm, so the day became a bit of a blur. The nausea slowly settled down and I was still hooked up to a drip.

Whether you stay in hospital overnight or longer, take some ginger tea bags to the hospital with you, as ginger tea has been found to be useful in reducing nausea, especially if you end up having chemotherapy or radiation treatment later on.

I was also hooked up to a catheter, which was inserted into my penis – otherwise known as Mr Percy/Mr Dicky/Willy/Johnson/member/one-eyed snake. The other end was inserted into a urine bag to collect what seemed like an endless flow of urine. This bag then had to be drained during the day and throughout the evening by the nurse. So, I was not moving around too much in the bed; it was difficult to get comfortable, and my ability to move was fairly restricted anyway.

At some point in the afternoon, the staff brought around refreshments, so I attempted to nibble on some dry biscuits and sip some pineapple juice; it seems that is useful in settling the nausea down. There was no dinner for me that night as even the smell of food put me off.

Whether you are in for robotic surgery or having 'open cut' surgery, take in a few flexible drinking straws, so that you are able to drink easily from the glass. Attempting to roll to the side or sit up can be difficult, as this involves the abdominal muscles, which will have been cut during surgery and they will be very sore.

Fiona rang me early that evening, and I struggled to sit up to get to the phone, again due to the abdominals not wanting to function. I became emotional and cried while talking to her – not really sure why, but it may have been the accumulation of events, and the reality of what had occurred was sinking in. That night I did not sleep well at all; I was feeling itchy from my chest down to my groin area.

Prior to the operation, a chest rash had been a problem over the years, even spreading at times to my scalp. Ever since my return from Vietnam in 1970, the rash had been there, flaring up depending on what my health was doing. It is irritated by heat, sweat, and any increase to my stress levels. I know I am not the only Veteran who experiences such rashes.

I attempted to give myself Reiki – this is a hands-on healing method that I have practised and taught for years – it seemed to work as I drifted off at times, but it was not a restful night. My hands became very warm doing the Reiki, which seemed to irritate the rash. So, Wednesday night offered a broken sleep and Thursday morning did not come early enough.

Finally, morning did arrive, and it sure had been a long night. The nurse suggested that I have a shower, but I felt the need to do a bowel movement. Before this could happen, the nurse needed to remove the drainage tube from the lower right side of my abdomen. She asked me to take in a couple of breaths and wiggle my toes as she slowly removed the tube. It felt rather weird, not painful, but a bit uncomfortable; anyway, it was out and she then put a small clip bandage over the wound.

This wound seemed to take the longest to heal, often feeling itchy, even twelve months later. The other incisions only had one or two stitches with a small clip bandage over them, including the one in the navel where the prostate was extracted.

Some months on, the scar in the navel became uncomfortable as new body hairs grew out of it, and at times it felt painful, as if there were needles pushing out – probably being the hairs coming through. That eventually settled down in the ensuing months. The nurse then helped me to sit up on the edge of the bed, and I quickly found out that the abdominal muscles still did not want to work.

Sitting on the side of the bed, I slowly tried to stand, and nothing wanted to function; legs, brain, there was no co-ordination happening. It was a weird feeling, knowing what I wanted to do and that it was just a matter of getting the body to respond, but at the same time, nothing wanted to move. I had to mentally talk to myself to get moving, and I was feeling washed out.

So with the catheter inserted in my penis to drain the urine, and the other end of it into the collection bag, I carried the bag as I slowly moved towards the toilet. I called the bag my '45', as it was in a similar position to where I wore my pistol when on guard duty in Vietnam. I was still wearing the theatre gown which, of course, was open at the back; now I know why it's called ICU!

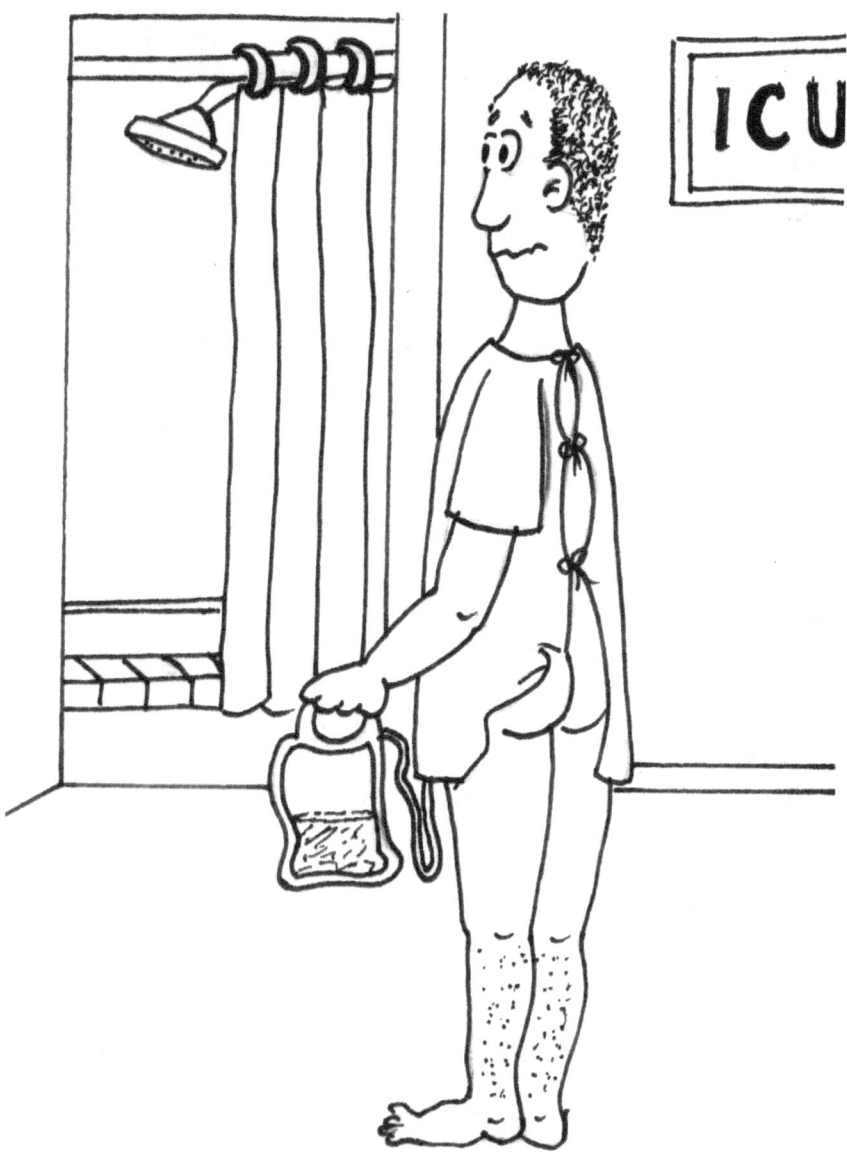

4. The Operation and the Aftermath

Thank goodness there was a hand rail on the wall of the toilet to grab onto, so I could lower myself onto the toilet. I sat and sat. There was some wind and rumblings, but not much movement down below for a while, but eventually some watery stuff came forth and I did feel better for that.

Some of you may find bowel movements take a while to return to normal; you will have to be patient for some time to come, maybe months in fact. Also, I found having thongs to wear instead of slippers in the hospital makes it easier, especially for the shower.

Getting off the loo was interesting as I had to focus on my legs, especially my thighs, to push me up slowly off the toilet seat, and using the hand rail to pull myself up, as the abdominals were very sore – all while hanging onto the urine bag.

Now I took myself into the shower, where the nurse helped me take off the gown while I juggled the urine bag to avoiding knocking the catheter. This was certainly no time to be worried about being exposed in all my glory, and I was sure she had seen plenty before.

So, sitting on a seat ledge, I slowly showered myself with the hand-held shower head, and the water felt good on my body; albeit, a very slow process.

I eventually ended up back in bed, but sitting on the edge, as breakfast was being delivered. As it had been a while since I'd eaten, I opted for a small quiche, eating slowly so as not to reactivate any nausea.

Guess who forgot to take the ginger tea bags into the hospital?

Tony Costello appeared again, and we chatted about the operation. Apparently, it had gone well, with no external cancer detected in the seminal vessels or in the margins of the prostate, so at this stage all was well. A blood test for PSA would be done later on to check whether there was any residual PSA present.

Fiona came to take me home. The nurse showed us how to attach the night bag to the day bag, which was strapped onto my thigh above the right knee with an elastic slip-on gauze-like bandage.

I think the night nurse was tired because, as she

demonstrated attaching the bag, it was upside down; so she had to get another one. We were given two overnight bags to use, and reminded to ensure our hands were clean when attaching and emptying the bags.

With paperwork in hand, we asked the nurse to sign off on the paperwork as the Department of Veterans' Affairs (DVA) was covering the account, since prostate cancer is accepted by DVA as being due to service in South Vietnam. We then went downstairs to finalise the paperwork, where we were given a bit of a run-around, and I was in no fit state to be going backwards and forwards; no one seemed particularly sure about who signed what.

So, if you are a Veteran and having a prostate operation (or any other operation), ask the hospital's Patient Liaison Officer, or the Veteran Liaison Officer, to help out. In my case, neither was available, nor were they even aware I was in the hospital, yet this was noted on the admission forms. Not impressed about that.

We went home by taxi – an easier option than attempting to park around the Epworth. I slowly eased myself into the front seat of the taxi and the driver asked if I had injured my thigh.

The driver was Indian, and he was completing his studies in Melbourne, so I launched into my prostate spiel about men keeping healthy and why that's important, for most of the trip home. I don't think he was even aware he had a prostate or what it does; most young blokes don't either. So, he was a bit more informed about his prostate, and hopefully he does take care of himself.

The operation was a watershed for me as it was not what I had been expecting, having come so far with active surveillance – some ten years. In the days to follow, while recovering, and every time I attempted to sleep, or I awoke up in the early hours of the morning, all the events, incidents and experiences pertaining to my recovery kept shouting at me to be written down.

So I started to write down thoughts, ideas, feelings, and emotions, not in any particular form, but just to get them out of my head so I could refer to them later when I felt like attempting to put them into some sort of book.

5. Let the Healing Begin

Back home, Thursday, and having an upstairs bedroom made for an interesting climb. I didn't know which leg to use first, as I could feel my abdominals wanted to be involved as well and they were very sore. Anyway, it was a slow climb up and down the stairs. I had been told by my physiotherapist that I would have to lie down for at least two hours a day to rest, as I was still recovering from the operation – I found I was sleeping a lot.

For some time I didn't feel like eating much and, as I was not going to be doing a lot of exercise right away, I was very wary about putting on weight. I was still experiencing a feeling of nausea floating around, so I only ate if I felt hungry. I suspect this nausea may also have been a reaction to the anaesthetic. In fact the nausea took a while to go and tended to hang around for some time after the operation.

I only had the catheter in for seven days, so I decided not to bother going out socially. On the Friday after the operation, I attempted a short walk with Fiona, but only got about fifty metres when I started to feel very tired and unwell. I realised I didn't feel right, so we turned around and went home.

I have spoken to, and heard of, some men socialising quite soon after the operation – including a friend who went out for dinner while wearing his catheter. Remember, everyone is different and will respond differently to this operation or other treatments. Personally, I was not interested in going out. I found that I became quite tired by the afternoon and had to have a nap.

The attachment of the urine collection bag to my leg – I call it my '45' – was certainly an experience in itself. The bag had to be emptied regularly. It had a small snap-lock at the bottom to let the collected urine out. Due to my abdominals being so sore, I found it very difficult to bend over to empty my '45', so this is where true love comes in.

Fiona and I got up close and personal. Fiona came with me to the loo to unlock the bag and empty it. Being a small loo, it was a bit of a juggle for us both to fit in there, making sure we didn't knock the catheter at the same time.

Make sure your hands are clean; the last thing you need is an infection.

We made sure that the '45' nozzle was aiming into the bowl before it was released, and unlock, aim, fire! It's a good idea to use your hand to flatten out the bag to ensure all the urine empties out. Then make sure the nozzle is locked back into place – and don't forget to wash your hands.

It's amazing how much urine is produced during the day, and I had to keep the fluids up as well; at least 6-8 glasses a day, so it did not take long to fill the '45' throughout the day. Night time was a different scenario, as the night time bag (holding 2 litres) was attached to the day bag to collect the excess urine overnight.

The night bag had a tube which was inserted into the nozzle of the '45'. You need to place the night bag into a bucket, and it's a good idea to put an old towel into the bucket, just in case there is a spill! The bucket I used was yellow, so I called it the 'Yellow Peril', after the infamous Melbourne sculpture of the same name and colour.

I chose a square bucket as it's easier to move with your foot along the floor, if you have to, and less likely to tip over

5. Let the Healing Begin

than a round one. Now, where to position the bucket on the floor next to your bed for the night?

You might well think, towards the end of the bed; but that is where you will put your feet down if you get up in the night, straight into the bucket. Not so great! So, place the bucket on the floor, about in line with your waist, and against the bed so there is no stretching of tubes. There will probably be nightly visits to the loo, as I discovered, for bowel movements, so you will be carrying the bucket with the night bag in it.

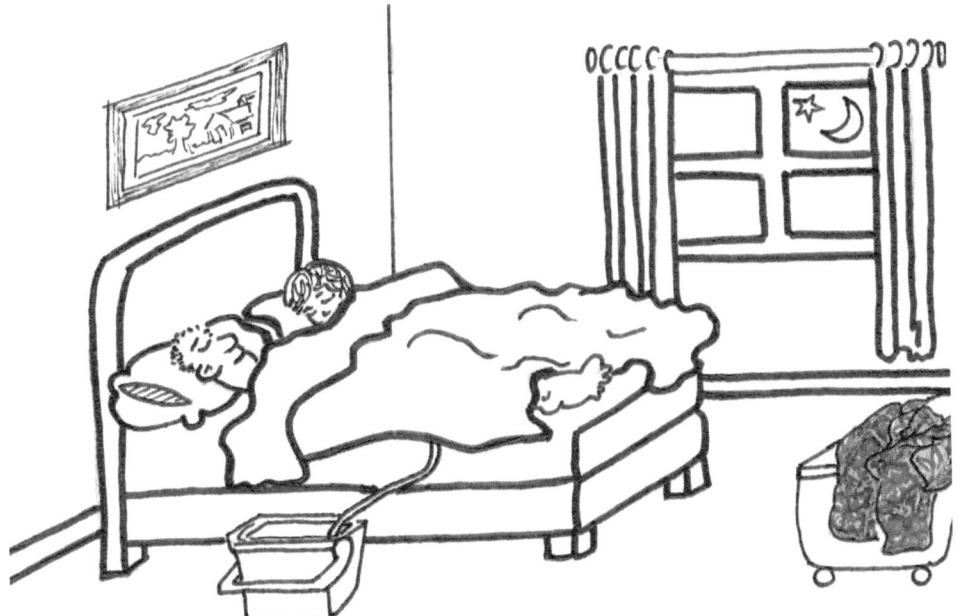

This was another interesting part of the recovery process; I found that my bowel movements took some time to return to normal, or what I called normal for me at least (one bowel motion a day). So, often over the next seven nights I would wander off to the loo carrying the 'Yellow Peril' and sit, waiting for movement down below. Luckily for me, we already had a hand rail on our toilet wall, so this made it easier to lower myself on to the seat and to raise myself off again. The abdominals were still not functioning properly.

It is important that you don't push or rush the bowel

movements. Your physiotherapist will have instructed you on how to breathe when attempting a bowel movement. It's important that you don't try to hurry things up; this is a good time to sit and contemplate the universe! After three or four days, I found that I was able to bend over and undo the nozzle to release the collected urine myself, although the abdominals were still feeling tender.

Having a shower for the first three or four days proved an interesting experience; I found it easier to sit in a plastic chair in the shower recess. I initially took off the crepe bandage that held the '45' to my lower thigh, and held the urine bag while Fiona washed me – especially my back and shoulders – which felt really good.

I even had Fiona dry me off initially, as I was still feeling very tired and just didn't feel up to showering and drying myself. I must say that, as this happened; I felt somewhat like an invalid and thought that this was not how I wanted to be in the future.

Eventually I left the '45' attached to my leg and sat in the chair to shower myself, but towards the end of the seven days, I was standing and showering, and then changing the wet crepe support for a dry one – which held the '45' – after showering. I also washed very carefully around the catheter to remove some small dry residual blood and leakage, which seemed to have an odour – well, at least I could smell it.

Sleeping during this initial period felt disjointed; I could not roll onto my side because of the catheter attached to the overnight bag, so I didn't always sleep through, even if I didn't get up to go to the loo. Often I would wake up after an hour or so, and my mind was up and running with thoughts about the operation, how I was coping or not, whether all the cancer was gone and a myriad of other thoughts and concerns, including how I could put these thoughts into a book.

My other concern was the removal of the catheter at the end of the seven days, due to my previous experience of that very painful extraction. I had spoken to a friend who, in the previous twelve months, had also undergone radical prostatectomy, which involved him being cut open due to

5. Let the Healing Begin

the aggressive nature of his prostate cancer. He informed me that there was no pain at all when his catheter was removed. At the time, I still needed to be convinced otherwise.

I knew that the catheter I had in also had a small balloon within its structure, but I didn't know much else. So, about eight days later, Fiona and I were back in Tony's office for the results of the operation, and to have the catheter removed.

Tony informed us that it was all clear; there was no residual cancer, all the margins were clear, with no seminal vesicle involvement – these are small glands attached to and located towards the top of the prostate. The extra prostatic extension – the tissue surrounding the prostate – was removed to ensure the cancer had not spread and that was also clear. So, there was no need for additional therapy like radiotherapy or chemotherapy.

Great news for both of us, and Tony was very happy with the way the operation went and with the results. I was given a copy of the pathology report, which stated that the total prostate involvement was 1.43%, tumour volume was 0.5cc, with the peripheral zone tumour being 0.55cc, including an index of 0.33cc, all of which appeared to be rather small. Basically, this meant that the tumour volume was small, but it was sitting around – inside the edge – of the prostate.

As most of the cancer was in the peripheral zone, it may not have taken long for it to go 'walk-about'. Lucky for me that I had that biopsy back in January, otherwise I might have had a different outcome in twelve months' time.

I can remember looking at the report later and thinking, "so why did I have it out when there seems to be such a small amount involved? Maybe I could have dealt with the cancer after all." But I needed to remember that it was in the peripheral zone of the prostate and that it might have gone 'walk-about', and then I would have been in deep shit!

Tony also discussed the use of Viagra™, but more about that later in the Entertainment section. Fiona and I then went with Helen to have the stitches and catheter removed, which I was still not looking forward to. Helen did assure me that it would be okay, so I dropped my trousers – I seemed to be having a number of women looking at Mr Dicky – and hopped onto the couch.

I was wiggling my toes, breathing and waiting for it to come out. Helen explained that she would deflate the balloon and then remove the catheter. Suddenly, it was out, with no pain and only a slight sensation. I am still surprised at the ease of the catheter's removal; obviously things had improved over the years. I think Helen had done this before! Fiona was in the room at the time and later said I was looking pretty apprehensive as Helen did her thing.

Now Helen helped me put on pull-up absorbent pads, a bit like the nappies that toddler's wear – now I did feel like a baby! But it was a relief to be without the catheter. Fiona and I decided to celebrate by going to our favourite coffee shop and then to do some shopping.

Before you go to have the catheter removed, check that the clinic will have pads available, or take your own. This was something I did not do and, luckily for me, Tony's clinic did have a supply.

The idea for coffee was good, but I had forgotten that I was still constantly leaking. After about 30 minutes, we left the café, and did a quick shop. But I discovered that my pad felt very heavy in the crutch and I had a wet spot on my pants; they were a light colour, so the wet spot was very obvious, bugger!

There was no bladder control at all, something I completely forgot about. Even though the pad was a number 3 – the heavy-duty one – it was very wet and uncomfortable, a good lesson for the future.

If you do end up wearing pads for some time, avoid light coloured pants just in case the pad does leak. Dark pants don't show the leak mark so readily.

These pads can be ordered directly from Independence Australia, rather than hunting for them in a chemist or supermarket. Luckily for veterans, DVA will cover this expense if it's related to an accepted disability.

There is also a Federal Government scheme called

5. Let the Healing Begin

Continence Aids Payment Scheme (CAPS), which can assist in the purchase of pads. The Continence Foundation of Australia can be a good source of information about CAPS, and all things to do with incontinence.

During the following months, the number of pads I needed over a 24 hour period slowly decreased. In February, I used around seven of the number 3 pads –heavy duty ones – over 24 hours, and by the end of March, I was down to five over 24 hours.

There are several different types of pads that men can purchase. Initially, I obtained what I thought would be useful, but it turned out that they were like nappies, in that they were very bulky and had side tabs to hold them together and keep them up.

I was pretty annoyed when they were delivered, as I felt they were not practical at all, and totally inappropriate to wear under pants. They may be okay for much older men who are continually incontinent and unable to control their bladders at all, or able to look after themselves, but I felt like a bloody baby trying to wear them.

Initially, dealing with the company to get the pads exchanged proved a bit frustrating, as it turned out that every time I wanted a different type of pad or 'level' of protection, I had to get the doctor or urology nurse to authorise the script.

So, a word of advice, if you can, plan ahead. When you need to change the level, advise your medicos early of your changing needs, and order them in advance so you will have the pads ready when you need them.

Eventually, I had the first batch of pads exchanged for the pull-up briefs for men, level 3 size; much more practical, not as bulky, and easily worn under shorts or trousers.

Again, every man is different and individuals may find that they are continent quickly after the operation, don't need the pads for very long, and are okay with buying their pads from the chemist – each to his own.

The weeks following the catheter removal, I found I was getting up two or three times during the night to change the pad as it became full. This was accompanied by the sensation that I was going to have a bowel movement. This is where you have to be patient, as you sit and wait for the movement down below to happen. Sometimes there is a bowel motion and other times just wind and little else. What's that old saying about a barber's cat? – 'all piss and wind'. That's how I sometimes felt!

Also, you have to remember not to push or strain when attempting a bowel movement, as this will weaken the pelvic floor muscles. If you feel a sneeze or cough coming on, remember to tighten your pelvic floor muscles so there is no leakage from your bladder.

Getting up during the night can play havoc with your sleeping pattern, so be prepared to take a nap during the day. I often did this by actually laying on the floor with my legs on the sofa and my head on a pillow; this position flattens the back out. I found this helped to take pressure off the bladder, and you can do your pelvic floor exercises whilst lying down like this.

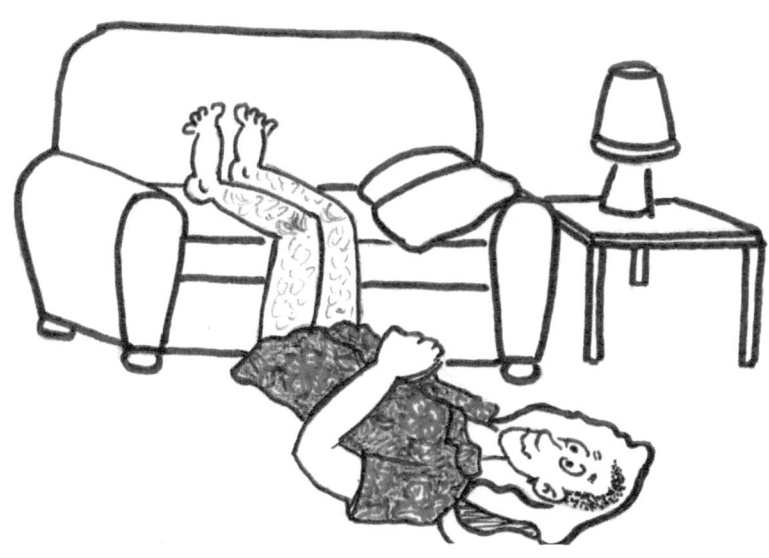

5. Let the Healing Begin

For a few weeks or so after the operation, I had a queasy, nauseous feeling, which tended to put me off my food, so that by the time I would get up, do a meditation or give Reiki to myself, it was late morning. I often ended up having brunch and then not eating again till dinner that evening.

I was now drinking up to two litres a day, but the nausea or queasiness would return from time to time, or whenever I had overdone things by standing too long. This happened at a couple events, like the Air Show at Avalon and again on ANZAC Day.

Over the ensuing months, there were visits to see Rebecca, the physiotherapist. I was keeping charts of the volume of fluids I was drinking, and measuring how much urine I passed at each visit to the loo. I was also weighing the pads to see how much urine I was voiding into the pads.

These measurements showed how much the bladder capacity was increasing, and also the amount of time between visits to the loo. She was also following up to see how I was going with the exercises, and adding new ones to the mix so that the pelvic floor was being strengthened constantly.

On some days, my bladder capacity would be up to 400mls, and it would be up to two hours between visits to the loo; then there would be a day when I just kept going to the loo and my bladder capacity went down. Thankfully, those days were becoming few and far between.

Even though I wore pads at night, I still woke up with an urge to go to the toilet. Sometimes the pad was fairly damp due to the constant leakage, and I would need to change it for a dry one. At least by going to the toilet to pass urine, this was giving me a sense of some control, in that the body/mind connections were working – waking me up to go to the toilet. There continued to be little bowel motion and, if there was, I had to be patient, by sitting and waiting for the motion.

The strange thing about waking up to go to the loo was the mind's involvement. I would have these very realistic dreams of going to take a pee, and I would wake up there and then. One minute, I'm asleep and then I'm awake and needing to go to the loo. This still goes on, except when I get to sleep right through the night, which is a blessing as I wake up feeling so much better afterwards.

Sometimes I was not sure whether I wanted to pass urine or have a bowel motion; the best way I can describe the feeling is that it felt like pressure from within the lower abdominal area (bladder/bowel) and would spread from the scrotum around to the back passage/buttocks area. In fact, it was a very visceral feeling, and I would describe it as feeling like a cone spreading with its base down over these areas. These feelings lasted for a couple of months or so.

Interestingly, there was no real pain from the operation, just discomfort from the abdominals being sore, and a little shoulder-tip pain, for which I used heat packs. This is referred pain from the diaphragm, and related to the carbon dioxide used to inflate the abdominal cavity during surgery for robotic and laparoscopic prostatectomy.

For about a month or so after the operation, there was perineal pain; this occurs after robotic surgery and is felt between the back passage area and the scrotum. It was more noticeable when I went to sit down, so I took to having a cushion on the seat. Suggested treatment is to take oral anti-inflammatory drugs, but I never did and, in time, the pain went away.

Over the following months, the pad usage slowly reduced, as did the pad size. From the initial number 3 – the pull-up briefs – I graduated to a number 2 pad, which is less bulky and just inserts into your jocks. Later, I moved on to a number 1, which is a lot slimmer; of course, the pad's capacity to absorb urine is lower with each decrease in size.

The incontinence pads are worn inside a man's jocks, or briefs. They cannot be worn in boxer shorts. The pads have two vertical adhesive strips which adhere them to the inside front of the briefs. I took to adding a smear of glue from a UHU stick, along the front horizontal area of the pads so that they stayed stuck to the right place in my jocks. I did this because, as the day wore on, this part of the pad would bunch up and move down the inside of my jocks, making it uncomfortable and a fiddle to deal with when attempting to take a leak.

When wearing the number 2 pads, I discovered that, as they became full, the weight tended to drag or stretch the crutch of the jocks, so it might be an idea to use any older jocks that you might have and wear these around home. When I was out and about, I found it useful have some newer jocks to insert the pad into, as these newer jocks are more likely to support the pad, rather than being stretched in the crutch area.

Leakage was another matter, for there were moments when I would go "oops, there goes a spurt of urine", over which I had absolutely no control. This would often happen when standing for too long, or when I was sitting for a while.

This would be frustrating at times and I would have to remind myself that the incontinence would heal in time, but as the middle of 2011 came around, there were still days when I just seemed to go to the loo to pee all day, or I seemed to be continually leaking.

I found this very emotionally difficult to handle and I would become angry. Sitting on the toilet, I would cry about the situation I was in, wanting it to be over and done with, to stop bloody leaking, and there was that feeling of not having control over what was happening to my body.

This was a good reminder to keep up the daily exercises for the pelvic floor. Even twelve months on, I still found that standing too long could increase the leakage rate, and I needed to ensure that I wore a pad if I was going to be out for any length of time, just in case.

There are two examples which come to mind where I was on my feet for too long in the first few months after the operation. The first was when I went to the Air Show at Avalon with a mate on a trade day. We arrived at about 9.30 a.m. and I was on my feet all day, except for lunch, until about 4.00 p.m.

I wore the pull-up briefs, which can absorb a fair bit of urine, but I ended up going through three pairs of briefs that day. Thankfully, there was no waiting at the toilets; however, it was bit of a hassle getting shoes and pants off in a small cubicle so I could take off the pull-ups and put clean ones on. The Air Show was great, especially because we were able to get fairly close to the aircraft, and talk to the pilots and crew, which made up for the inconvenience of the toilet visits.

That night I was tired, but it was over the next two days that I felt wiped out and just not feeling right; it was similar to how I felt during the first two weeks or so after the operation. I had overdone it by being on my feet for too long, forgetting that I had been through a fairly major operation. Boy, did I leak for those two days; the bladder and pelvic floor were not happy! And the nauseous feeling returned for a day or two.

ANZAC Day was another occasion where I initially thought that I might give it a miss, being only two months after the operation. There continued to be days when I just felt tired and out of sorts, with some days of little leakage and others not so great.

In the end, I decided to go and take a spare pad. I wore a number 2 pad that day. Luckily, on that ANZAC Day, the RAAF Vietnam Veterans stepped off on time and, when we finished our march behind the Shrine, we headed off to the restaurant opposite the Shrine in St Kilda Road. As the day wore on, the leaks started and I eventually filled the pad quickly; thankfully, I had the spare available to use.

The following day, I did not feel flash at all. I felt wiped out and was leaking all day. I felt slightly ill, a bit like how I felt in the week following the operation. I guess I thought I would be okay – wrong on that account. In fact, a good friend and fellow Vietnam veteran, Stan, had suggested that it might be wise not to march due to the after-effects of the operation. I did not listen to his advice and, as ANZAC Day drew closer, I thought I'd be okay and didn't want to be watching the march from home.

So, a good lesson is to listen to your body, as it can take time to recover, physically and mentally. Yes, every man's recovery will be different. I am still surprised at how quickly some men go back to work; maybe it's mind over matter!

5. Let the Healing Begin

I do know that, for 2011, it took me most of the year to heal and get over the operation. What added to the mix was that I was not working, as I had closed my clinic in April 2010 to concentrate on completing my Graduate Diploma in Counselling. I felt that, as I was improving, I should be working and yet I wasn't finding anything that I might apply for; so I was putting pressure on myself to be out there working. And I think I jumped back into my volunteer work too quickly.

This sort of self-imposed pressure does not help the healing process in any way. If you are still working, give yourself plenty of time to heal and use your sick/personal leave; you don't get any medals for coming back to work early. Again, every man is different and will respond according to his own physical and mental wellbeing at the time.

Drinking too much coffee and alcohol will irritate the bladder, as will carbonate-fizzy drinks. So, for a while, I took to drinking decaffeinated coffee, and I found that I wasn't enjoying alcohol either for some time. An occasional drink did help with the sleep, but if I had two drinks, I ended up with a slight headache the next morning. Of course, as one gets older, the body's ability to handle alcohol changes, and if you are not drinking enough water, you can become dehydrated, and alcohol adds to the problem.

I found that I became hyper-sensitive to the smell once there had been any amount of leakage into the pad. The pads do have an odour-control built in to them, but I found the odour – stale urine and sweat – would then permeate the crutch of my pants via the jocks. Also, there was increased sweating in the groin area, which added to the odour mix.

It reminded me of my visits in the past to aged care facilities to visit clients. This in itself may not seem a big deal, but I thought that if I could smell the odour then others could too. My wife told me that she couldn't smell anything; I guess I am just very conscious of my body smells.

Even today, without wearing pads, there seem to be small leaks occurring. Sometimes I am not aware of this, and then I notice that my jocks have a spot that is slightly dampish and, of course, I can smell that. This is something I am still coming to terms with, and it makes me even more determined to continue with my exercises so that I am not incontinent.

I also became aware that the crutch of my pants/jeans seemed to take on a slight odour from my jocks, due to some leakage. So I took to spraying that area with a eucalyptus spray to reduce the odour. I guess I am a bit fussy about my clothes, and cannot stand any stale or smelly odours of any sort in my clothes; hence my spraying them if there was even a hint of any odour.

I eventually rediscovered Johnson's Baby Powder, now made with corn starch along with Aloe vera and vitamin E; this certainly helps with the odour. What is also useful when washing your jocks, jeans or pants, is to put about a dessertspoon of bi-carb soda into the wash, or in the final rinse; this helps to deodorise the washing.

So, if you are facing surgery, start on your exercises as soon as possible, see a continence physiotherapist for specific exercises to do pre- and post-surgery and, if possible, work on your fitness by walking, bike-riding, swimming and the gym, if it grabs you. The fitter you are, the better your recovery will be.

Also, learning some stress management strategies, or a simple meditation, will assist to bring some calmness and balance to your being and help you face the coming challenges.

Around April 2011, I decided that I had had enough of the pull-up pads, and put a level 2 inside my jocks to wear to bed at night. This proved to be more comfortable, but as one who never wears anything to bed except a tee shirt in winter, it still was a bit annoying feeling 'closed in'.

In the first six months or so of wearing the pads, I developed an itchy rash of sorts around the perineum to the rectum area. I put this down to a combination of sweat and urine, and the area concerned being closed in by the pads. I used an aromatherapy-based cream that Fiona made up for me to deal with the itch, but it wasn't till I stopped using pads at night that the itch finally settled down.

Later on I remembered about wet-wipes that are used on babies, so I started using these after a bowel motion; this quickly resolved any itchy rectum issues.

In May, I made what I thought was a good psychological decision not to wear any jocks or pads to bed at night, and it felt great, a sense of freedom. It also felt particularly good to snuggle up to my wife without anything preventing that skin to skin feeling.

When I got up in the mornings, I wouldn't put on my jocks to walk around first thing, as I had previously done for some time (it's okay, the neighbours couldn't see anything, I think!). Again, it was a mental thing, a challenge to be able to hang on, rather than leaking into a pad or the jocks.

It was a matter of overcoming that psychological barrier of 'you might leak' thinking. Of course, there was the occasional slip-up but, on the whole, it was another hurdle that I overcame, and it felt good to be moving closer to being completely continent eventually.

I continued to see the physiotherapist for exercises, to check on my record-keeping for the bladder, and how much urine I was holding and passing. Some of the exercises were becoming more difficult, but the thing is to persevere if one wants to become continent.

I know from talking to some men, that the exercises did not seem to work for them. I don't know whether that was due to them not doing the exercises regularly or not doing the right ones. Of course, some men are continent some weeks after the operation; I don't know how that happens, but we are all just very different I guess in how we heal.

There are some useful books and DVDs which I have mentioned in the resource section that provide further information in this area.

As for the bowels, I was having plenty of fibre, including my wife's home-made minestrone soup, which in the past would certainly get me going; not so this time. I took to adding plenty of fresh garlic to dishes, or garlic powder, and coating salmon in cayenne pepper, which did make some difference to the bowels. Yet, twelve months on, the bowels were still taking their time to return to what I consider to be normal for me.

I have since read that there are two signals that can activate the need to pee and, especially after the operation, one has to be able to recognise them. One is the full bladder feeling, and the other is actually a 'urine coming' signal from the urethra. If one keeps responding to the urethra signal, then the bladder never gets to fill to its capacity.

Another point is that if the bowel is full there may be pressure exerted onto the bladder area from the bowel, leading to a feeling of needing to take a leak. In fact, it's a bowel motion signal, so one has to be aware of the signals you are getting from below and maybe it's a case of sitting on the toilet seat to see what is actually happening.

To overcome the urethra signal, you need to do ten quick clenches or pull-ups, as if you want to stop yourself from having a leak or passing wind (farting). By this time, you should be able to do them anyway, so these exercises are for the 'just in case' moments; the more you practise them, the longer you can go between leaks.

And they do work; although it did take me a while to get a sense of which signal was which. The exercises do reduce that urge for a leak and this helps to build up the bladder's capacity to hold more urine. I even practise them in the car when I am waiting at the lights.

There could be many reasons for this urge and, given that this may be the only signal some men get to void initially, it may be best to pay attention to the urge and go to the toilet. It is probably a good idea to discuss your urges and what they actually mean with a specialist continence physiotherapist. They should be able to help you know whether to go or whether to continue with your clenches. As always, get professional advice.

Even if you are not having problems with your prostate or bladder at the moment, being able to do these exercises will help to tone up and strengthen the pelvic floor muscles for later in life.

6. Wake-Up Calls, with the Advantage of Hindsight

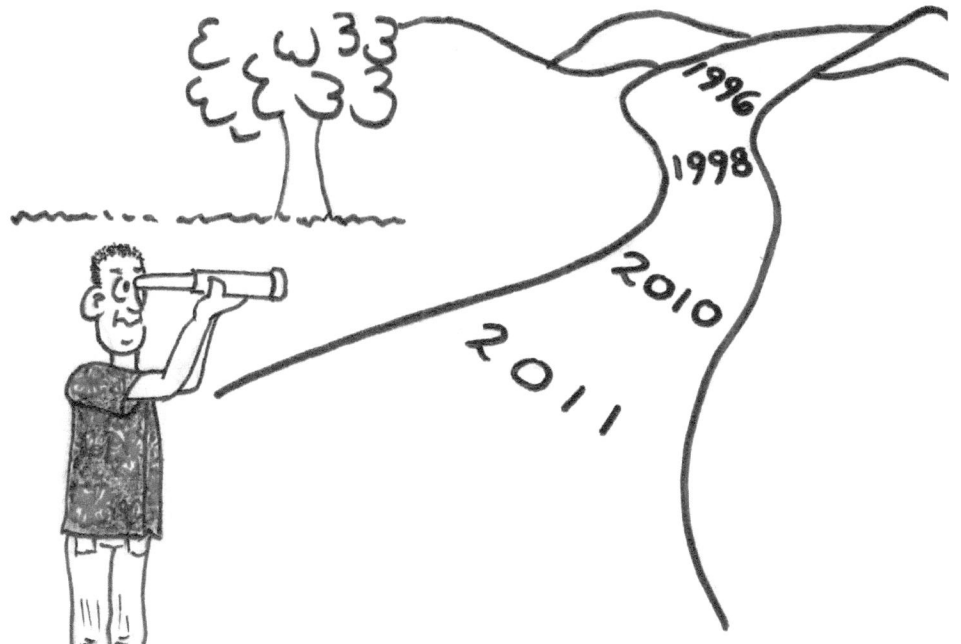

The following events that make up part of the history of my prostate journey were, on reflection, like taps on the shoulder to let me know that I was not being as vigilant as perhaps I could have been with my health.

Maybe the ongoing stresses that I encountered over a period of time were starting to impact on my immune system and its ability to deal with any infection or disease that was occurring within my body; like getting regular cold sores.

Being a Vietnam Veteran may have contributed to the prostate problem, as veterans have a higher rate of prostate cancer than the general Australian male population. As stated earlier, no two men will have the same experiences, symptoms, or even outcomes.

If this story at least encourages men, their partners and families to become more aware about prostate issues, and of taking care of their health, then it will have proved useful. I hope it will help any men who do end up with prostate cancer to make the best choices possible for their specific set of circumstances.

It all started around 1995, at the time I was living in Albury-Wodonga. I started to have problems with broken sleep, getting up two or three times a night to visit the toilet, and then being tired at work the next day. As I was a natural therapist, doing a lot of body-work and remedial massage, I needed to be focused during the day with clients.

Aside from the nocturnal visits, I was also experiencing deep lower abdominal discomfort, just above the pubic bone area. I eventually went to my doctor who decided to do a digital rectal examination – DRE. The prostate gland felt firm to him and he suggested I see a local urologist for a further examination.

After another DRE with the urologist, and in light of my problems with the water-works, the urologist decided to do a trans-rectal ultrasound of my prostate. This involves placing a probe up into the rectum to view the prostate; which I found very uncomfortable, to put it mildly – no anaesthetic. Later on, he did an inspection of my bladder with a small tube up the urethra, via Mr Percy; again, not pleasant.

It was discovered that I had prostatitis, inflammation of the prostate, for reasons unknown. The ultrasound showed small calcium-like deposits within the prostate; again, due to causes unknown.

So a course of antibiotics was prescribed to deal with the

prostatitis. At first, I baulked at having to take the antibiotics, thinking I could deal with this naturally. Wrong on that account; prostatitis requires treatment and, if not dealt with properly, can become chronic (I did take the medication).

If you do have any pain or discomfort in the lower abdominal area, or into the perineum/groin area, go to your doctor and get this dealt with ASAP.

Because the prostate felt firm on examination, the urologist decided to do a further trans-rectal ultrasound biopsy of the prostate, via the back passage – the rectum. This is done to take tissue samples from the prostate for examination by the pathologist to check on the state of the gland.

It was something I was not prepared for, as there was no local anaesthetic. It was bloody uncomfortable, to say the least, and I counted the clicking of the needles as they were fired from the probe, through the intestine wall and into the gland to collect the prostate tissue.

I felt uncomfortable for a day or so after this event, and emotional for some reason; I am not sure if it's because I was not ready for the procedure or not really advised about what to expect. I actually felt violated in some respects. I have read that some men don't find it too much of an issue; again, we are all different, and react according to how we feel and experience at the time.

Now the bladder had its own issue, as the urologist discovered that there was an obstruction or growth partially over the neck of the bladder where it empties into the urethra. So that accounted for the numerous visits to the loo! The bladder was not emptying fully. I had also not been feeling well for some time, sort of off-colour, and perhaps it may have been due to the retention of excess urine.

A week later, the pathology report came back with a PSA score of 0.5, which is fairly low. The tissue samples were taken from the left and right base (bottom of the prostate), mid, and left/right apex of the prostate, with four of the sections showing benign prostatic glandular elements.

Some sections of the tissue were showing atypical glandular elements, but no definite evidence of malignancy.

The prostatitis eventually settled down, but over the following years it did return intermittently and, now that I knew what the symptoms were, whenever the prostate started acting up, I went straight to the doctor for treatment.

Consequently, I had an operation on the bladder to remove the obstruction and spent a number of days in hospital, hooked up to a catheter to drain the bladder. On the morning of discharge, I was woken up at about 6 o'clock for the catheter to be removed. I was not sure what to expect, but the expression 'pissing razor blades' should give some idea of the pain I experienced, even if only briefly.

Recovering from this operation took a while, and the bladder-continence issues did heal, but it was some time before any sense of normality returned. After the operation, and in the following years, my need to go to the toilet took on a different aspect. Now I needed to be aware of where the toilets are, and I didn't seem to be able to hang on as long as I used to. For the next couple of years, I had regular check-ups and the PSA was still low. Following this procedure, there was never any mention of seeing a physiotherapist for pelvic floor rehabilitation.

In 1998, I moved back to Melbourne with my partner at the time, and to continue university studies. My studies didn't work out as planned, so I started working at the Hilton on the Park spa complex from 1999. In early 2000, I realised that it had been nearly two years since I had had a prostate check-up, so I got a referral from the urologist I saw in Albury to see a colleague of his in Melbourne. The blood test for the PSA was done.

I was admitted to the Austin Hospital to have the biopsy procedure done. This time, I was given a couple of suppositories to place in my back passage in order to clear out the rectum. This enabled the ultrasound to form a clear picture of the prostate for taking the tissue samples, and reduced the possibility of infection.

My partner at the time accompanied me at the hospital while I waited for the suppositories to work, as she had to drive me home after the procedure. Not having used suppositories before, I was not quite sure what to expect, but it didn't take long for a reaction. Very quickly I was sitting on the toilet, and there was plenty of movement happening down below.

I was eventually wheeled into the theatre for the procedure – again, no anaesthetic. This time, I felt a bit tense, laying on my side with legs drawn up into a foetal position.

I was told there would be six to ten needles fired into the prostate to take samples. This time, I decided to count them, backwards, to take my mind off the event. A nurse who was in attendance, very kindly held my hand while the procedure was carried out.

The procedure was finished and I was wheeled back to the ward to recover. My partner was waiting for me and we eventually drove home. I felt uncomfortable and a bit out of it, and ended up having a couple of days off work.

A week later, I rang the urologist for the results and it was not good; the biopsy had come back positive with a Gleason score of 6 (it was 3+3), with a PSA of 10.9, meaning a grade of T2. I was pretty pissed off with the results. I was angry, annoyed and felt like I was in no man's land. That evening, while preparing dinner, I put on some rock and roll, cranked up the music, opened a bottle of red and still felt bloody angry; not that drinking was going to help, but at the time it seemed a good idea.

I went to see the urologist to discuss the results. He wanted to remove the prostate, but I was not that keen. I wanted another opinion, and time to consider my options.

I was able to get an appointment with Professor Tony Costello, head of urology at the Royal Melbourne Hospital. We met and he ordered a review of the prostate tissue samples taken; the score was now a 5, but Tony also wanted to remove the prostate. Again, I wanted time to see what I could do to create some changes. Tony suggested I take Selenium and gave me a prescription to get some.

In the meantime, I browsed the web to see what other men had done and there was plenty of information out there, but it was all about working out what does and doesn't work.

To compound things, the relationship wasn't travelling well, as I had been having an affair and my partner found out. So, there was infidelity on my part and the added stress of what was happening within the relationship. It had gone pear-shaped, to say the least.

I was feeling backed into a corner, and considering that I am a Natural Therapist and Reiki teacher, there was no way I was having my prostate removed without doing everything possible to create healing of some sort.

Over the coming months, and with Tony's support – albeit reluctantly, as he was keen to pop my cherry – I embarked on changing my diet, undertaking a short fast, taking the appropriate supplements and giving myself plenty of Reiki. I even spent a week with another Reiki teacher for additional treatments to sort out what the hell was going on with my body and how I got to be where I was. After a couple of months, Tony performed a further biopsy, and the results still showed that cancer was present, although with a low score.

Tony did not want to wait too long and picked a date to operate, even though I was still resisting. All this occurred in 2000 and that meant radical surgery, which at the time meant being cut open or what I call 'open cut'. At this point, I was donating my own blood for the operation, as there is often blood loss with this type of surgery.

In the meantime, I was still looking on the web for information, although it never occurred to me to see if there were any men's support groups around, as there are now. I did ring the Cancer Council in Melbourne to get any other information they may have had. The operator suggested maybe having some Reiki; I told her that I was a Reiki teacher!

When looking at various medical websites concerning prostate cancer, the statistics for this type of operation looked at things like incontinence, erectile dysfunction, complications and even death on the operating table. Funnily enough, the death rate – very low – was not my main concern; it was the incontinence and erectile dysfunction that loomed out at me.

Tony assured me that, over twelve months, the incontinence would get better, as would the erectile function, due to my age (49 at that time) and health. I was still working on myself and it was getting closer to the operating date. I kept thinking that I could not be doing the type of work I did and lose my prostate to cancer!

As the operation date approached, I asked Tony to do one more biopsy, just in case there had been a change; I didn't want my prostate cut out only to discover there was no cancer in it.

Tony agreed to do one more biopsy, without anaesthetic, but gave me a couple of Mogadon™ prior to the procedure, to relax me. So I sat in the waiting room and started to drift off, sort of. The biopsy was done and a week later I called Tony's office for the results, but he was tied up and the receptionist said he would ring back.

After a couple of phone calls back and forth, eventually I was told that the tissue samples were showing benign, not cancerous! Tony wanted to see me ASAP – I bet he did. My partner and I went to see Tony to discuss the results, which were a bit perplexing, as there did not appear to be any logical answer for the turn around.

Now, for something out of left field. About two weeks before the biopsy, I had a dream in which I was told – by a cousin in the dream – to pray for divine intervention, which I did. Leading up to that point in time, I had been giving myself regular Reiki, taking supplements, and dealing with a relationship breakup.

So what worked to create the healing? To be honest, I am not really sure; maybe it was a combination of everything that I was doing. I think that, in certain situations, changes occur and we don't really know what causes the change. Maybe I was given a second chance, as my Reiki colleague said, "And don't stuff it up, as there might not be another chance!"

7. Dressing Percy

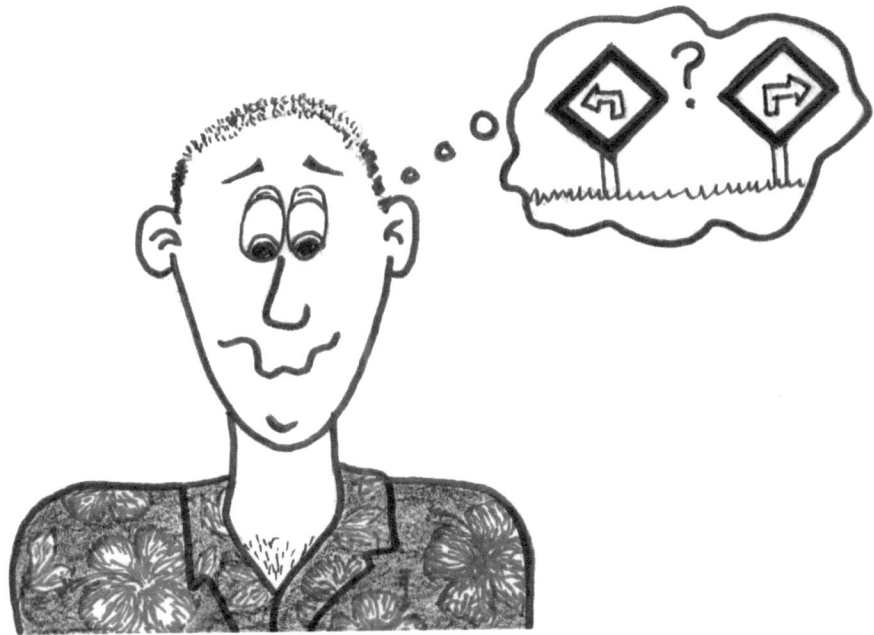

Have you heard the following phrase, in which a tailor, who is making a suit for a man, asks "Which way does Sir dress?" It refers to how Mr Percy hangs, to the left or to the right. Your answer, either being left or right, then influences how the tailor adjusts for that when making the trousers.

Since birth, my right testicle was undescended; it had been sitting up in the lower abdomen until 1972, when it was finally operated on and removed. Fiona therefore nicknamed my left testicle 'Han Solo'.

Now, being the owner of only one testicle, the left one, I naturally dressed to the right. So, after having a catheter in for seven days and inserted into the '45' – the bag – on my right thigh, I felt that Mr Percy dressed even more to the right.

As a result, I found that, when wearing pads of all sizes, this had an interesting effect on the way that urine emerged; it seemed to be always to the right area of the pad. Sometimes I would adjust Percy so that he aimed into the middle of the pad, but this wouldn't last for long, as he would drift off to starboard again.

Now another phenomenon occurred, due to Mr Percy's 'eye' being pressed up against the pad. It seemed that whenever I took a leak, the 'eye' was partially closed and this affected how the urine came out. This continued for some time, even when just wearing jocks without a pad.

As most men know, at the end of a leak there is often a dribble or two that require a few shakes to clear, as sometimes there can be some residual urine still sitting in the system – inside the urethra. So, just when you think you're finished, there's that inconvenient spurt to wet your jocks or pants front.

Before I explain how these flows may come out, here are some tips on how to possibly reduce those embarrassing moments; best practise these at home initially.

Firstly, I had read an article in *The Age* newspaper some time ago about the pros and cons of standing versus sitting to take a leak. Sitting on the toilet to pee, and leaning slightly forward, was found to empty the bladder more effectively. I now do this most days when I am at home. If I am out, I generally stand to take a leak. It is also important not to rush or force out the urine, as this tends to weaken the pelvic floor muscles – the same goes for when you go to do a bowel movement. So, be prepared to sit, relax and go with the flow of your body's natural rhythm.

The second tip is one for all men, of all ages, whether or not they have had a prostate operation. Every man will benefit from the following simple technique, which helps to ensure there is no residual urine sitting in the urethra and waiting to sneak out when you least expect it.

This technique is done while standing and involves taking your middle finger – I use my index finger along with my middle finger – and placing them up behind the back of scrotum, where it joins the area of the perineum.

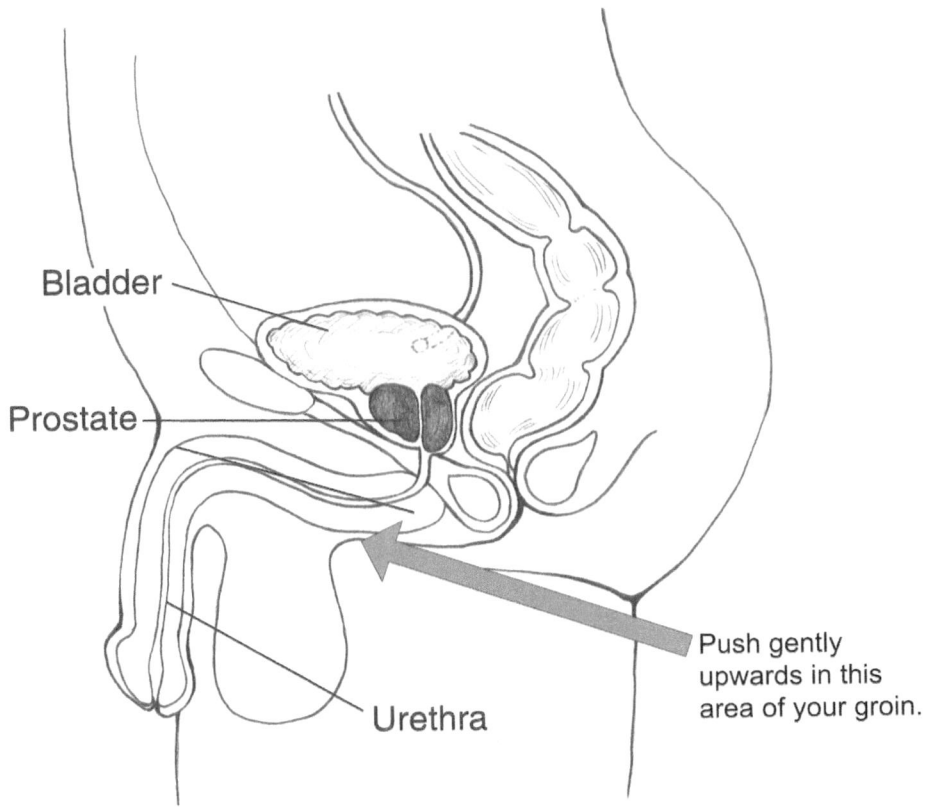

You do this after you feel that you have emptied your bladder. You gently push upward into this area of the body, which creates pressure on the urethra, encouraging it to release that last bit of urine sitting in the urethra end of the penis. I believe this also called "Milking the urethra".

I still give Percy a bit of a shake again, just to make sure. I also grab a piece of toilet paper to dab Mr Percy afterwards, as I often find there is still some residual urine just sitting there waiting to escape.

This may take a bit of practise, but it is not difficult to master. You may need to push upward into the back of the scrotum a couple of times, and give Mr Percy a bit of a shake afterwards.

Now, concerning the 'eye' of the penis. In my experience, during the first six months or so, I found that when I went to take a leak the 'eye' was partially closed; consequently, the urine did not come out in one steady stream.

I also found occasionally that, because Mr Percy was shorter after the surgery, the hairs in the groin region would become stuck across Percy's eye. As a result, when I would go to take a pee, the flow would come out at different angles, as described below. My solution was to trim (very carefully) the hairs around Percy to reduce the likelihood of a rogue hair getting stuck across Mr Percy's eye!

Mr Percy is somewhat shorter due to the operation, so he can be a bit difficult to grab onto and point due South. There is now some excess skin around him, and it can be a bit slippery; more on that later.

So, here are some types of flow that you may experience if you don't give Mr Percy a bit of a gentle stretch before taking a leak; which, in itself, can be difficult because of the urine sitting in the urethra ready to flow.

There is the 'spray' shot – all over the seat/bowl – of course, you always pull the seat up first – down the sides of the bowl, and possibly down the front of your pants as you attempt to point Percy due South.

Then there is the '45 degrees' shot – this occurs when the urine shoots out either left or right, as Percy's eye seems to be half-closed. This means the urine hits the wall, the spare toilet rolls, maybe the side of the vanity unit, or anything else within range! A bit embarrassing if using someone else's loo, or in a public toilet!

There are several reasons why Percy is now shorter; one is that, when the surgeon cuts out the prostate, a small portion of the urethra will be removed and this appears to having a shortening effect on the length of the penis.

The other reason is that the nerves that lie around and under the prostate are damaged and traumatised to some degree.

7. Dressing Percy

There are two groups of nerves involved in this area; one lot contract to create a pulling effect that shortens Percy – similar to the shrinkage that occurs to men who have been in cold water. Then there are the lengthening/relaxing nerves; unfortunately, it's the shortening nerves which are reducing Percy's length.

If you are sitting down to take a leak and you are not pointing Percy down into the bowl with a finger, then you may get the following effects.

There is the "oh shit" 'straight-over-the-top' shot – you are sitting down to take a pee and again, you forget to point Percy due South, but this time the urine flow goes straight over the top of the seat and either hits your pants, shoes, or the floor. If the flow is strong enough, it can hit the door as well.

Now, if you are standing up in a public toilet and the urine shoots straight out, that may not be such a problem. But if you are taking a leak at home or at a friend's place, then it means this shot goes Bulls eye and hits the toilet seat cover, possibly sprays everywhere, and runs down the seat cover.

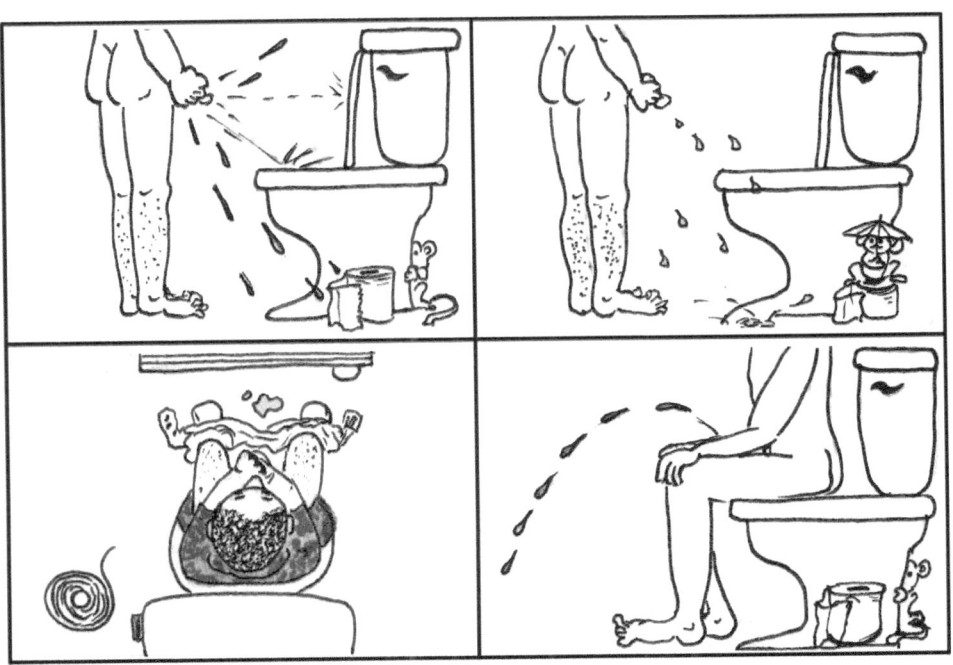

The 'under-cover' shot is a variation of the above shot, where instead of going over the top of the seat, Mr Percy shoots straight and level to underneath the seat and splashes back onto your groin, or runs through the gap of the seat and down the front of the bowl, or into your pants.

The last type I call the 'laser' shot – similar to the '45 degrees' shot, this occurs when you go to point Percy into the bowl and the eye is partially closed. The urine shoots out in all directions, and if you have been hanging on for a while, there will be urine hitting everything in sight!

And just to add to the fun, as you attempt to aim him, because of the extra skin that results from his shortened length, he can be a bit slippery. So, as you try to point him due south into the bowl, he can slip out of your grip and keep spraying everywhere except down!

My way around this predicament was to place my first finger on top of Mr Percy, and the middle finger below him, in a scissor-type position, directly behind his head. This gave me better control over pointing and direction, and you can gently stretch him. Of course, you may already do this; so much the better.

As I live in Sandringham, I was missing walks to the beach and swimming, so towards the end of March, Fiona and I would drive to the beach – I was still not sure about walking far with the pads I was wearing due to the constant leaking.

Once we got to the beach car park, I would slip the pull-ups off and put my speedos on. We would then walk down to the beach and into the water. As I stood there in the shallows, it felt so good to be back in the salt water. Of course, I was still leaking, but it felt so much better doing it into the water rather than into the pad.

I walked along in the shallows up and down the beach and, after a couple of visits, decided to see if I could swim. Unfortunately, as soon as I took the first two or three strokes, my abdominal muscles started complaining, as they were still very sore. So I had to be content for a while with just walking in the water. At least it was exercising my legs. By the end of summer, I was able to start swimming to some degree, although my fitness had really dropped off.

I eventually went to the local heated pool to swim, but it does take a few months or so for the abdominal muscles to heal. I also noticed that, with the regular exercises to strengthen the pelvic floor muscles, the lower abdominal muscles were becoming tighter, and I could feel them respond when I started swimming.

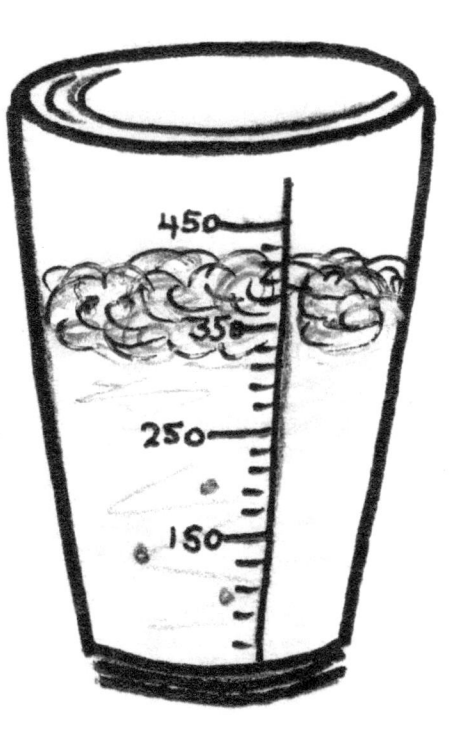

8. The Measuring Cup

In the months that followed the operation, I measured how much urine I was passing at any given time. I used a plastic tumbler produced by DVA which showed different standard drink measurements on the side. I made additional marks on it to cover the different volumes of urine that I passed. This tumbler held a maximum of 425mls (light beer), but there was room for about another 20mls.

Even when I got up in the middle of the night to have a leak, I had to pee into the glass to measure how much urine the bladder was holding. I had to note the time, date and volume. This proved rather amusing as sometimes the colour looked a lot like light beer, and at times I even produced a bit of a head – frothy – on top of the urine.

It was a good day if I had held off for an hour or so, and was able to produce a volume of around 425mls plus. The chart I filled in showed time, volume, pad changes and the wet weight – urine leakage – of the pads, so this gave a good overview of progress in the months following surgery.

Throughout the months of recovery, I had to keep up my water and fluid intake, as well as keeping track of how much fluid (and what sort of fluid) I was drinking each day (and recording the time and volume of fluid passed). I was looking at having to drink at least two litres of water each day, along with coffee and anything else. You might think that, with all that fluid, one would never stop leaking, but keeping the fluids up helped to increase the bladder's capacity to expand and hold more.

Keeping track of my fluid intake meant I was more aware of what and how much I actually drank. I also started to notice a difference within myself whenever I didn't drink enough fluids, especially water.

I have come across research suggesting that, when a person thinks they are hungry, they are actually thirsty; so by keeping a bottle of water or large glass handy, you can easily keep yourself hydrated. You may then find a reduced need to be snacking all the time.

It seems that the latest method of working out how much water you need is determined by your weight, and of course the type of work you do, either inside or outside.

Coffee and alcohol will dehydrate you so, for every drink of either, you will need to have a glass of water; but too much water will flush the system too much, so it's a matter of balance.

9. So Many Problems Solved

Almost a year after the operation, my bowel movements were still no better, although the continence continued to improve. I had even taken to swallowing some Senna tablets to see if I could get extra motions happening, but these only partially helped, and I didn't want to become reliant on them.

After visiting the doctor, I got a referral for a colonoscopy, just to make sure there was nothing else holding up the works. I decided to have this test because I was over 60 and I had been doing the annual faecal occult blood test every two years, which had always proved to be negative.

If you are over 50, it is recommended that you consider having a colonoscopy, which involves having a tube – with a small camera – placed into your rectum and up into the large intestine, to see if there any polyps or growths that shouldn't be there. This is highly recommended, especially if there is a history of bowel cancer in the family; in my case there was no such history.

The day before the procedure, I had to drink two litres of warm fluid that tasted like lemonade, and take some Senna tablets. I should mention that for most of the year I was only eating two meals a day, and, if there was lunch, it was usually light. Because of this, my body did not have a lot of waste products to move through the bowels.

Eventually, early that evening, after drinking all the liquid, there was movement at the station, down below, and I had to be quick! This continued for the rest of the night and, to some degree, the next morning. Not that there seemed to be much in the way of substance, if you get my drift; mostly water and wind. Well, at least I got a good clean-out.

The procedure was performed at a local day hospital and my mate Ken dropped me off, as you are not allowed to drive on the day of the operation. I did one more quick visit to the loo at the hospital, and then into the operating room. You are put out to it with a light general anaesthetic, and that certainly worked quickly enough. Waking later, I was told that everything was okay, except for a couple of polyps – which were removed – and a small haemorrhoid.

The polyps were sent off to the laboratory, but were found to be clear. Of course, this procedure does muck around with the bowels and they can take a while to return to normal. Again, I was not eating a lot, and I found my bowel movements/signals to be quite subtle.

Making Progress

A year after my operation, the continence issue had improved but there would be an occasional day when I would leak, and if I was going to a meeting or would be on my feet for a while I would wear a level one pad, just in case.

There would also be days when I seemed to be going to the loo more than normal to take a leak. I associated these frustrating days with not doing my exercises regularly.

I have now added some additional exercises to my pelvic floor regime. Basically, these involve doing sit-ups, but first contracting the pelvic floor muscles, and then pulling the belly button/abdominal muscles down towards the floor to flatten the lumbar area. Then you pull on the abdominal muscles to lift your neck and head off the floor. This, in

9. So Many Problems Solved

turn, strengthens the pelvic floor muscles. Doing plenty of walking, running – if you are able – swimming and other activities mentioned in the book below, all add to improving the pelvic floor muscles.

These exercises came from a book called *Conquering Incontinence - A new and physical approach to a freer lifestyle,* by Peter Doran. I certainly found that, after a while, these additional exercises made a difference to my incontinence issues, so that I was able to hold on longer. By doing the ten quick clenches, this gradually did make changes to how my bladder functioned.

As Peter says in his book, "never ever give up on doing the exercises"! Persevere, persist, talk to the physiotherapist – especially one who is an incontinence specialist – to find out what else you can do; of course it can take time to return to normal, and every man heals differently. Even doing specific abdominal exercises will assist in strengthening the core muscles surrounding the pelvic floor muscles.

At a good friend's birthday lunch, I caught up with Dr Eric Dowker, Chiropractor, whom I had known for a long time. I mentioned my experience with the prostate, including the incontinence and erectile dysfunction. Eric also uses kinesiology – muscle testing – so he did some quick tests on me then and there, and discovered that I was out of balance, badly!

I made an appointment to see him. That first visit went for an hour. Dealing with incontinence, erectile dysfunction, bowels and the ongoing cold sores I was experiencing, I had tears of relief – probably due to a release of tension, and a realisation that I needed to have seen Eric sooner. I did feel so much better for the treatment.

It was a relief to get myself and my body back on track, with the first noticeable response being later that afternoon – my incontinence practically did a 180 degree turnaround. I didn't have that ongoing feeling every half hour or so of needing to take leak.

Over the following weeks after the visit to Eric, I was lasting longer between visits to the loo, and my bowels also started to return to my version of normal.

I made further visits to Eric to make sure my body was functioning properly – the incontinence and other issues. I believe that Eric's treatments have certainly made a big difference to my healing – mentally, physically and emotionally.

Interestingly enough, when I discussed the bladder problem with my physiotherapist in the months following the operation, she explained that it was possibly due to the bowel, for if it was full, it applied pressure to the bladder – because of the bowel's close proximity to the bladder – thus the feeling of needing to take a leak so often.

So, if you do have the operation, be aware that the bowel may impact on how your bladder functions for some time after the surgery. Your bladder function will also be affected by how consistent you are with your daily pelvic floor exercises.

10. What We All Want to Know

This chapter is difficult to make a start on, partly because of the subject, but also as I do not want to imply that other men's experiences will be the same as mine were after the operation. The following is only an account of my experiences, which may prepare the reader for their own adventures.

This chapter also demonstrates that a loving, caring partner, who is ready to understand the after-effects of the operation, and willing to engage in sexual intimacy, can encourage healing on all levels for both concerned.

Prior to the operation, I had been told by the urologist that it would be useful to take Viagra™ as there was some evidence that, by doing so, it would start acting on the nerves located around the prostate to assist in the healing. This was important both prior to the operation and after, especially to get the blood flowing into Percy.

So I bought a packet of Viagra™; $89.00 later and with only four blue tablets, this was certainly an expensive supplement. Because the script wasn't authorised by DVA initially, I had to pay up-front. Fortunately, I was later able to be reimbursed by DVA after supplying the script and authorisation number.

For any DVA clients, remember to ask your GP, urologist or practice nurse to ring DVA for an authorisation number for the script; that way you will only have to pay around $6. If you go down the track of having to inject yourself, get your doctor to obtain an authority from DVA for the injection material and the needles. The number of needles you buy will determine how much you pay for them.

Initially, I was advised to start with a quarter of a tablet; they are 100mgs, so I was to take 25mgs each day, on an empty stomach to aid absorption. Food and alcohol will interfere with the uptake of Viagra™. Magnesium supplements will also interfere with Viagra™ uptake.

Cutting the tablets was interesting, so here is a tip: as the tablets are in a blister-type pack of four, you gently pop the back of the individual tablet but leave the seal still attached. Then take a sharp knife, place the blade face down on the top of the tablet, and push down firmly to cut the tablet in half. This way the tablet doesn't shoot off, as it is still in the blister pack. You can repeat the process to cut a quarter tablet.

There is of course a cutting device you can buy from the chemist, which is much easier.

Something rather interesting happened after taking the first quarter tablet of Viagra™, remembering that this was before the operation. So I had taken the little blue pill late morning, with no breakfast up to that point. I noticed that Mr Percy felt rather full and that I had a partial erection, without any other stimulation. Fiona was home, as she was not working at the time, so we decided to make use of the situation, if you get my drift – that's right, we had sex. It didn't take much to get Percy up and running with stimulation!

There was a downside to taking the little blue pill initially – there are several potential side-effects from using this medication – and for me that was a headache and some flushing in the face. Over time, the headaches settled down, with just the occasional flushing. The two other oral medications are Levitra™ and Cialis™, which act in a similar way; you may not get a full erection, but some fullness, and with stimulation you can move towards a stronger erection.

All three medications are called PDE 5 (phosphodiasterase type 5) inhibitors, and all work on increasing blood flow to the penis. Professor Rashid advises that all have their own side-effects, such as facial flushing, headache, nasal stuffiness, lower back pain and indigestion. My own experience was the headache, facial flushing and some short-lived indigestion. Other possible effects are blue-green vision or light sensitivity with Levitra™, and, for Cialis™ there can be lower back pain and thigh pain.

You may need to persevere with one brand of oral medication for up to ten doses, or use another brand for a while to see which works best for you.

If, in time, there seems to be little response, then you may need to move onto needle injections into your penis; that is, after the operation and if the tablets are not working for you at all. There is also the vacuum device that can assist in giving you an erection.

These options will have to be discussed either with your urologist or your GP, so as to decide on the best protocol to use. Every man is different and will respond accordingly to the various medications. The injectable medications are either Trimix™, a liquid which needs to be made up by a compound pharmacist, or Caverject™, which is contained and blended within the injecting unit prior to injecting your penis.

If you haven't already bought Bettina Arndt's book, *What Men Want in Bed*, then I suggest you do so, as you will get to read about other men's experiences with the different medications and devices available, including vacuum pumps and penile implants.

Leading up to the operation, I continued to take the little blue pill. After the operation, I was advised not to take the tablet for at least a week or so, and then to go back to taking it, as part of rehabilitating Percy.

11. Trial, Error and Success

A week after having the catheter removed, I was back at the urologist's rooms to see Helen, the urology nurse. She was to administer an injection into Percy; then I would return the following week and, under her supervision, inject myself! This was the bit I was not really sure about. These injections are intended to get blood and oxygen into Percy, and to help achieve an erection, so that there is less chance of scarring inside Percy in the long term.

So, with Fiona in the room, Helen showed us the Caverject™ injection needle, which has a prepared mixture within the syringe part of the device, so you can dial up how much you want to inject. Helen dialled up an amount of 5, and then explained how and where to inject into Percy. With me sitting on the side of the examination table with my jocks dropped, Helen gently took Percy in hand, and because she is right-handed, injected into Percy on the right side.

The needle is fairly small – it is similar to what a diabetic would use to inject insulin into themselves; it's a BD Ultra-fine syringe. The feeling of the needle being pushed into

Percy is similar to a mosquito bite, but with a touch more ouch, somewhat unpleasant. It looked and felt strange having this done so that I could have an erection!

I pulled up my jocks and jeans and was given an instruction card with diagrams so I would know how to do the injection in future. As we were about to leave, Helen said "You won't be using this when you get home" – referring to the erection that was about to follow – and told me that it would take about 10 minutes or so to kick in.

We had parked the car in Bridge Road, not far from the Epworth, because the visit was only brief. Also, because we did not know what sort of reaction would occur, I did not want to use public transport – I am so glad we took the car.

Fiona was driving and, by the time we had driven over the Yarra and down Punt Road, Percy was starting to react and I could feel an erection coming on. Half way home, I was feeling very uncomfortable, so I undid my jeans and sat sideways to give some space to the emerging erection.

By the time we got home, Percy was feeling somewhat painful. I lay down on the bed and examined Percy; he was looking very thick, swollen, decidedly erect but painful. Helen was right – there was definitely not going to be any afternoon delight! Although the shaft was hard, it felt very sensitive and uncomfortable.

I had been told that I could take some Panadol if the erection was painful, which I eventually did. I also tried walking around, in the hope that it might help to drain some of the blood away from the groin region. I ended up lying on the bed attempting to find a comfortable position to somehow reduce the painful feeling of the erection; however, by the time the Panadol kicked in Percy was starting to deflate, so to speak.

Of course, having an erection for too long, or having one that won't go down, is a risk. As described in Bettina's book, this condition is called Priapism; an erection that lasts longer than four hours is dangerous. This is a complication that leads to the erectile tissue being killed off, much in the same way that a heart attack kills heart tissue.

This condition needs to be treated medically if it lasts that long. Apparently, taking Sudafed can go some way to relieve the congestion of the erection. Of course, you do not want to be taking oral medication and doing the injections as well – that is definitely asking for trouble. So, after about an hour, the erection started to subside and I was thinking that the next time must be better.

On my next visit to Helen for supervised self-injecting, I related my experience from the last injection, so Helen decided to use the Trimix™ formula instead. This still involves injecting, but you draw up the desired amount of fluid – from a bottle – to be injected into Percy. Also, the formulation is different from the Caverject™ formula and there is less likelihood of such a strong reaction and side-effects. The Trimix™ formula is a combination of prostaglandin, papaverine and phentolamine.

I was feeling somewhat apprehensive about injecting myself, but a man's gotta do what a man's gotta do! And that is to keep the wife happy! So Helen showed me how to draw the liquid from the bottle and we started with about 40cc. The syringe holds 1ml, with measurements on the glass body of the syringe so you can determine how much you want to draw in.

I gingerly pushed the needle into Percy. There was a sting and then I injected the liquid in. I didn't really have time to worry about being watched by Helen, as I was too focused on getting the needle placement right. Fiona and I left to wait for the results at home. This time there wasn't such a strong reaction. In fact it was a bit of a strange one, as the swelling started at the base of Percy and gradually worked up to about halfway along the shaft. The swelling stopped there, creating a bit of a ring and then some slight swelling towards Percy's glans tip.

We had some foreplay and stimulation that afternoon, but it was like Percy was stuck between heading towards an erection and then losing interest. Now that I knew what would work, I went back to my GP to organise a script for Trimix™ and an authorisation through DVA to cover the payment.

This stuff is not cheap, so I am lucky that DVA does cover the bulk of the cost, although they also require written supporting clinical evidence explaining why I require the Trimix™. Well, hello, I have erectile dysfunction, meaning I cannot get an erection; I'm not injecting myself for fun!

I did persevere for a while with Viagra™, not only for the erections but also to get blood and oxygen into Percy, but even with a 100mg tablet there was no real erection, just some fullness, but certainly not hard enough to attempt penetration. As one of the men said at the support group, "It's like playing snooker with a piece of rope".

Now, for some good news. About 17 days after the operation, having taken a little blue pill, we decided to try our luck with lots of foreplay, stimulation and oral sex, and eventually I had an OMG orgasm. This orgasm happened without me having an erection, so the good news, gents and ladies, is that it can still happen!

Actually, OMG is a medical term – Oversized Male Genitals – not that it describes my present condition now!

I have in the past certainly had some amazing orgasms prior to the operation, but this one and the others that followed were to the point of being nearly unbearable, which up to this point in time I thought was not possible.

12. Consequences

Over the coming months, my orgasms at times verged on being painful and, in the early days, there was a small loss of urine – called Climacturia – when I climaxed. However, in my experience, the Climacturia effect didn't seem to happen after about six months, although it's a good idea to empty your bladder before the fun begins. I don't recall being told I might experience either of these problems after the operation. Nor do I recall being told about penile shortening.

It is important to remember that these are dry orgasms, because the vas deferens that carry sperm from the testes (and join the ejaculatory duct which runs through the prostate gland) have been cut, so they're either tied or clipped and the sperm have nowhere to go.

Strangely, in conjunction with the OMG orgasms, it felt at times like there was an ejaculation occurring. In fact, the pelvic floor also felt as if it was involved, so that added to the intensity of the orgasm, and to the feeling of ejaculation.

During some of these intense moments, I would be overwhelmed by the orgasms, and I was very aware of something happening deep internally in the lower abdomen/ groin area, as if there was some sort of ejaculation happening.

In time, the testes stop producing sperm, so you become infertile. Therefore, if you are younger and still want a family at some point in the future, you may want to look at the options of harvesting your sperm and freeze-storing it for future use. If you are single and do partner up again and want children, you may also want to consider this option, or even donating to couples who are having problems conceiving, via the IVF program.

At times I felt like I was totally part of the orgasm and, at other times, part of me was waiting for ejaculation to occur, with a sense that, on some level, it still was, even if it was internal. I suspect that there was some sperm movement happening as part of the orgasm, but presumably any sperm was disappearing somewhere inside the pelvic cavity.

In Bettina's book, some men talked about the intensity of their orgasms and I tend to agree that they can be very intense, to the point of being nearly unbearable. Again, I must point out that every man is different, and how you will react after the operation will depend to some extent on how sexually active you were prior to the operation.

As men get older they can take longer to become aroused, to get a full erection, and to reach orgasm. How often you have sex prior to the operation can also be a factor in your post-operative experiences. After the operation you may find you take longer to climax, and this is partly due to nerve damage from the operation.

Then it's a matter of whether or not you were waking up in the morning with erections – which generally occur throughout the night to keep Percy flushed with blood and oxygen. Your age and general health will also affect your erectile recovery. Another name for that erection on waking is a 'piss horn'. This may stop after the operation, and it's something I missed as part of my manhood! Although, in 2013, I occasionally woke up with a partial erection in the morning, but nothing like the old Percy.

Having discovered you can have an orgasm without having an erection, I also found the pelvic floor muscles wanted to get in on the act, so to speak, which they do when a man is having an orgasm. Something else that happened after the operation

12. Consequences

was that Percy's head (glans) became very sensitive, especially when I was inside Fiona, to the point of being unbearable or painful as the orgasm built up. This tended to depend on how long it was between being intimate with Fiona. Yet this feeling didn't occur as much if I masturbated.

Occasionally, I found there was a release of urine when I was having an orgasm, so it felt like I was ejaculating at the same time. That experience took the shine off the moment, so I made a point of emptying my bladder before we got physical. Once in a while, a sensation that I was about to leak at the point of orgasm still occurred, but eventually this feeling disappeared too.

Over the ensuing months, I took Viagra™ to get some fullness happening and, although it was never hard enough for penetration, it certainly added to the effect of stimulation as part of our intimacy and subsequent orgasm. I briefly took Levitra™, but didn't have much response, although I didn't try it for long.

I continued to use the Trimix™, slowly building up the amount of solution drawn into the syringe. This, in turn, produced some interesting reactions in Percy, from being partially full halfway up with some fullness near the tip, so he looked at one point like a 'bottle tree'. Other times he looked more like an hour-glass.

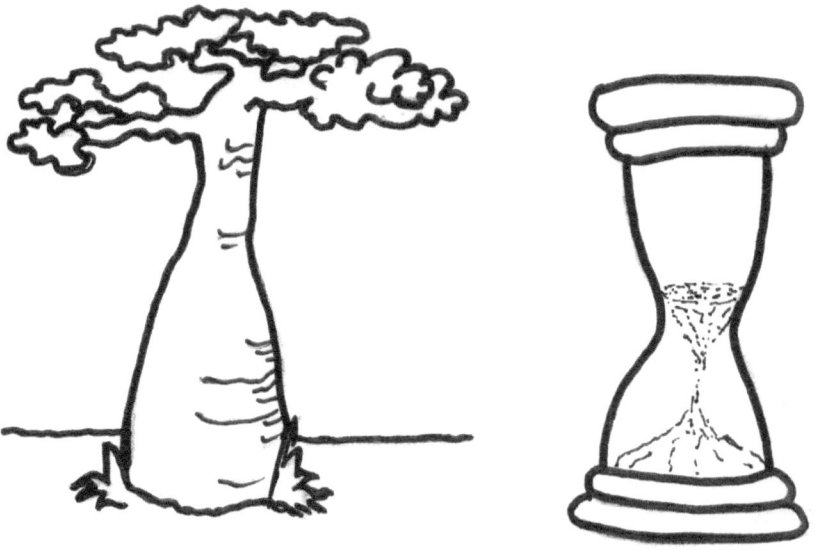

Of course, Percy was not hard or stiff enough for penetration, without a lot of persuasion, but again this added to the overall pleasure of being intimate with Fiona, who is very supportive in this area and we both gain a lot of pleasure from the closeness.

I find that I now take longer to reach orgasm and that Percy feels less sensitive to stimulation, sometimes to the extent that no response happens at all. The message just is not getting through to Percy.

It's as if there is a real disconnection between my brain and the nerves that activate Percy. I find I really have to work on the fantasy aspect – in my mind – to get anything happening down below. Fiona feels that I need to relax and not worry so much about what is happening, and that I am trying too hard.

For some time, I found this aspect frustrating; even when I masturbated in the shower, any reaction seemed to takes ages, with or without using Viagra™. There were moments during this process in the shower when I felt frustrated at not being able to reach orgasm. I felt useless and remembered how, in the past, masturbating to reach orgasm was so easy.

As hard as I tried and fantasised, there was a sense of something deep inside the lower abdomen wanting to happen, but nothing was responding. When I did eventually reach orgasm, I felt an emotional loss, of sorts, that I was not experiencing the full event. I felt frustrated at not being able to orgasm when I wanted to, in that it took so long to happen.

Again, I still had this feeling of no connection between Percy being stimulated and the nerves involved, absolutely nothing at all. My brain knew what was supposed to happen, but the messages were taking a long time to get through. I kept forgetting that it takes a long time for nerves to heal, and I had been told the erections could take up to two years to kick back in.

Also, since the operation, I found that Percy had lost some of his sensitivity, so that it took longer to feel like anything was happening or that an orgasm was going to occur. Again, this also depended on how often we had been having sex – longer between events meant that Percy was more sensitive – or if I was tired. The after-effects of the operation seemed, for me at least, to compound the problem.

When I did masturbate and the orgasm started to occur, it was fairly quick. The intensity of the orgasm was there (the OMG type) and that sense of relief afterwards. Strangely enough, initially, Percy was still not fully erect during this process. In fact, it was a weird feeling as Percy would actually become erect or full *after* the orgasm – talk about back-to-front reactions!

Having talked to a number of men who have also lost their prostates, I know they are no longer interested in sex, for one reason or another, especially if they are older. Still, for the health and wellbeing of your penis, you have to keep the blood and oxygen flowing in to prevent internal scarring.

The nerves that surround the prostate are damaged to some degree during the surgery, as the surgeon attempts to peel the nerves away from the prostate. These nerves are responsible for men getting their erections, along with being aroused mentally and physically.

For men who are experiencing any cardiovascular problems, these can also have an effect on whether you are able to gain an erection, or even whether you experience those nocturnal/early morning ones. If you cannot get an erection or do not get morning hard-ons, these can be signs that there might be a problem and you need to see your doctor.

13. Coming to Terms with Change

In the months following the operation, the incontinence and the use of smaller pads continued to improve, albeit a little slowly for me, and I continued to persevere with the injections. Building up on the amount of Trimix™ I would draw up into the syringe and inject into Percy, meant that his fullness was increasing. Then, six months later, there was a leap forward; after being out for the day, we decided on some afternoon delight.

We had considered sex the evening before; part of me wanting to do it, yet another part not wanting to use the needle. I sometimes wondered if my libido was waning, but I think it was the process of dealing with the after-effects of the operation and general stress which was dampening my desire. If I was honest, there was part of me that wanted to avoid doing anything involving the needle; it would have been great if the tablets were more effective.

I missed the spontaneity of the moment, of being able to have that sexual encounter whenever we wanted to; although I had noticed that, over the last few years before the operation, when I was a bit tired, I needed some help to get Percy up and running. Just being able to have sex whenever, so to speak, had now changed and, after reading Bettina's book, I found that there were other men who also experienced that sense of loss. There were some men who were injecting themselves and experiencing their penis return to its former glory, and expressing how that felt so good to them.

So, I gave the nether regions a clean-up, as I still experienced an odour after wearing pads all day, which is definitely not conducive to any sexual encounter. I prepared myself and, with some trepidation, I injected Percy. I have found that my anxiety occasionally causes problems. For instance, injecting into Percy's left side with my left hand, as I am right-handed, adds to my anxiety.

There are other times when I think to myself, we want to have sex, just go and do it. The discomfort of injecting is over in 15-20 seconds. What's that saying? 'Just do it'. Another saying that comes to mind is 'Stop complaining, you're an adult!'

Up to this point, I had been drawing in 40cc, so this time I drew in 50-60cc and then injected Percy. I jumped into bed with Fiona and began touching and caressing her; I could feel some stirrings down below, what I call tingles. I was expecting a full erection, but Fiona told me to relax, so we continued our exploring. We both became impatient, and Percy began to look pretty erect – without his middle appearing to have a 'belt-around-the-waist' look.

He was fully erect, but not as hard as he was prior to the operation; still, it was early days. So, after some extra lubrication, a helping hand and some persuasion, I was able to fully engage – penetration – and boy, did it feel good! With the sensation of being inside Fiona, I was feeling very aroused and, as we moved, Percy responded by becoming totally hard. Yay!

It had been some five months or so since the operation and I was finally able to be fully intimate with Fiona, and it felt fantastic. To have that full erection back and be able to do what I was doing before was such an amazing feeling, and Fiona wasn't missing out either. There was even a bit

13. Coming to Terms with Change

of serendipity involved, as that particular day was the anniversary of when I had proposed to Fiona!

It didn't take long for both of us to become even more aroused and, in turn, for me to reach an orgasm, which was very intense in itself, coming on quickly, sharp and almost to the point of being unbearable. It even felt like I was ejaculating, but of course I wasn't, as there is nothing connected and it's a dry run from now on. All the same, there was some sensation occurring down in the lower abdominal area and, along with the pelvic floor which also felt as if it was involved in the orgasm, that ejaculation feeling was pretty strong.

I had been told that I would get my erections back over the next twelve months to two years, and part of me believed that but, up to this point, Percy's reaction to the tablets had been so-so, and then the injections were not producing full erections. So I continued to increase the amount of Trimix ™ that I injected into Percy, which in turn produced a fuller erection, but it wasn't until I was actually inside Fiona and had become even more aroused that Percy would become harder and fuller.

Yet this feeling did not occur as much if I masturbated to get the blood flowing and to stimulate Percy.

In the first twelve months after the operation, Percy's head/glans was cold to touch and, at times, would look blue, so it seemed that little blood was getting through, or that damaged nerves were still causing problems. When manually stimulated, the head/glans would warm up slightly and Percy would take on a better colour. Often at night in bed I would hold onto Percy, or Fiona would, and this helped to get him warmer. Taking Viagra™ regularly seemed to reduce the coldness and blue colour; I can only assume that taking the other tablet medications may have a similar impact.

My internet research has discovered that this coldness happens, in part, due to the nerves being damaged during the operation, and they can take a while to heal. All the more reason, therefore, to keep stimulating Percy to get those nerves reviving and the blood flow moving. Yet, even 20 months later, there was some occasional blueness and coolness around Percy's head.

Emotionally, deep inside myself, I felt wounded. I had, in the past, heard other men talk of their experiences and even read about it, so I understood intellectually, but, like most things in life, until you experience the event it's all academic.

It's difficult to put into words just what I was feeling; mostly a sense of loss, due to being unable to have sex when we wanted to. The whole sexual experience had become so different, because it had to involve some planning. For example, if we wanted to go away, should I take the injection kit, or the Viagra™ with us? I had a sense of some deep emotional impact, but couldn't put words to it; was it just my manhood? Although, of course, there is more to being a man than being able to get an erection.

This was something that involved a part of my body over which I had no control. As for the incontinence, there were times I felt even angrier at my lack of control. I was persevering with the exercises, but there were days when I either leaked or continually needed to take a pee.

I would then get into a loop, thinking of what I could have done differently – again, this sort of thinking does not help the healing process at all. So, around August 2011, I decided that it was time I went back to counselling. I needed to get my head around what I was feeling, experiencing, and what I could do about it. There was also a sense of frustration about a number of things, but I couldn't quite put my finger on what it was. It was as if a door had been closed on part of my life, and now there were different physical, emotional and psychological issues for me to deal with.

On reflection, I think it would have helped me to have gone back earlier, but I thought I could get through on my own. Being a counsellor myself, I thought I could think my way through things - wrong! This idea actually came up for discussion in the counselling session, as in 'physician, heal thyself'. So, as a veteran, I went back to the Veterans'

Counselling Service to sort things out.

It was around the third or fourth session when, with the counsellor's help, I began to realise a few things about myself; such as how much I enjoyed flirting with other women and using my sexual energy, but also how much my identity was tied up with being able to be sexually active with my wife.

I realised that I, Alan, as a man, had so much of my own persona and identity closely linked to my sexuality. After the operation, I felt a deep wound, a loss of part of that ability to act sexually as I had in the past. Did I feel less a man? I looked the same physically, but my emotional sense of self required a re-evaluation.

I am not talking about running off and having affairs outside of my marriage – been there, done that in my previous marriage and relationships, and I'm not proud of having done so. Still, some part of me would wonder, 'what if I was single and had this operation? How would the whole sex thing happen then?'.

So it was this loss I perceived that I had to deal with, along with recognition that part of me had changed, and I would have to reinvent aspects of myself and function differently sexually. When I studied counselling, I had learned about the concept of 'disenfranchised grief', where there is ongoing grief over a particular loss. Most people are not aware of this, or it's often not acknowledged, either by the family, friends, or society at large.

I suspect that, in my case, and maybe for other men who have lost their prostates, there is a sense of loss and maybe a degree of disenfranchised grief because nobody talks about this to others. It's not like you meet up with your mate or some friends and say, "well, I'm not getting erections anymore and this is how I deal with it, or not".

I now had to face living and functioning in a different way in future. There were adjustments to be made on a number of levels; physically, emotionally and mentally. I was still a man, but I now had to function differently from the way I had prior to the operation.

When reading Bettina's book, I could see that couples certainly found other ways to deal with the change in being sexually active. As I keep saying, every man will have a different experience and outcome following whichever procedure he has. What is also important is the support that he receives from his partner, so this is where communication becomes crucial for both parties. There also needs to be an appreciation of the changes that have occurred, and willingness to experiment to see what works.

There are men who are single when they have this operation, as well as men who are gay, or bisexual. Who do they turn to for help with sexual matters, or for emotional support? That is something I am sure requires attention from the medicos and relevant organisations.

My light-bulb moment

Now for something a bit different. It was back in June 2012, on a Saturday night when there wasn't much on TV. Fiona was upstairs doing her genealogy research, so I decided to pick up a book I had been reading for a while. It's called *The Brain that Changes Itself*, by Norman Doige, MD. Lots of interesting information about the neuroplasticity of the brain and the way that changes can occur.

Picking up from where I had last read, I backtracked a bit to page 239, where the author discusses a case study about a patient undergoing psychotherapy, looking at dreams and their importance in analysis and, in turn, their relationship to the plastic changes within the brain. It goes on to discuss the patients who are haunted by recurring dreams of trauma and wake up in terror.

As these traumatised patients get better, their nightmares become less frightening. Now, you are probably wondering what this has to do with prostate cancer and recovery.

I had a light-bulb moment! For as long as I can remember, since serving in Vietnam, I have had ongoing nightmares of one kind or another, mostly war-related scenarios and mostly around Vietnam. During the last ten or so years, these nightmares had increased in frequency. Some of them were pretty scary and, from time to time, I would wake up from them not wanting to go back to sleep. There was no pattern to them; they could occur when there was a bit of stress in my life, or even at relatively stress-free times.

As I continued to read, past events came flooding back; pieces of the jigsaw puzzle began to fall into place, as I now perceived what those dreams may have been trying to tell me. The 'message' was that, on a deeper level, my body was under attack internally, specifically within the immune system and the prostate. Yes, the PSA readings had been low for some time, but, over the preceding 18 months, the levels had slowly gone up. When I had that last DRE, the prostate was firm, the biopsy result came back positive, and the rest is history.

The point now is that, since the operation in February 2011, and up to the completion of this book, there have been no nightmares of any significance. If I was to give my nightmares a score – with 10 being worst – prior to the operation, most sat around 8-9. After the operation, for at least four or five months, there were none; occasionally I had a dream of being back in the Air Force, but nothing like the type of dreams I'd had before. It was only in the latter part of 2012 that an occasional nightmare would occur, but only on a scale of around 4-5, or even lower.

So, I am suggesting that the stressors I was experiencing of all types, including financial survival and taking care of myself, had been a struggle for some time. There were others of a personal nature, but that's another story. All these experiences were hammering away at my immune system long-term, which is not helpful to anyone's health and wellbeing.

The nightmares represented to me that my psyche was under attack and, ultimately, my immune system, leading to my prostate being compromised. Well, that is a bit long-winded, but that's how I interpreted my reading of that particular chapter.

I realise that I am influenced by my background in counselling and natural therapies, but it made logical sense to me. Why else would the prostate cancer come back after all these years, given that prostate cancer is generally slow-growing?

My reading of that specific chapter of that particular book that night was an epiphany for me, so I wrote down my thoughts there and then, rather than waiting until later when I could get back to my book. There had been a multitude of feelings, emotions and thoughts, and it suddenly felt like a weight had lifted off my shoulders. I felt as if the dots had been joined, at least for me. There was also a sense of emptiness, filled with 'if only' thoughts: if only I had listened to the dreams, taken more care of myself, then I wouldn't be where I am now!

This awareness seemed to produce more questions than answers; more 'what ifs'. Would it have changed anything at all? I will never know, but that night I certainly pondered the 'what ifs' a lot. Since then, I have had to let go of those thoughts. It's a bit like the fork in the road – I made my choices and took this direction and, if anything, it has given me a better appreciation of what other men, and their partners, have gone through. It has also given me some authority to be able to speak about such events in the future.

14. A Wife's Perspective – Over to Fiona

At the outset, I would suggest that partners hold on tightly to their sense of humour and realise that they're in for a long, interesting journey.

When Alan's urologist informed us that Alan had prostate cancer, we both thought he was joking; his manner wasn't what you would expect under the circumstances. The shock was considerable when he told us he was serious and that Alan's cancer was 'aggressive'. My instant response was to agree with the urologist that surgery should proceed ASAP – Alan wasn't so sure.

I won't go through the worry, stress and fear that I felt when Alan went in for surgery. I will say that good friends are pure gold at times like this.

When Alan came home from hospital with his catheter and its accessories, we rounded the next learning curve. The nurse who instructed us in catheter use was very tired and consequently mucked things up. She didn't have time to go revise her instructions, so she just told us to do things back-the-front from the way she had shown us.

Alan couldn't manage to bend over enough to manage his catheter himself, so trips to the toilet were very cosy to begin with. Squeezing two adults into our very small toilet is a challenge in itself.

Thankfully, we employed plenty of humour right from the start. "Point and shoot" was the terminology used – once we worked out how to actually get the catheter into emptying mode. When Alan regained his ability to bend slightly, he was able to empty his catheter himself.

We took photographs of Alan in all his post-surgical glory – stark naked, but adorned with his catheter and its 'holster'. I think he felt quite proud of his new war wounds, but it wasn't pretty.

Another fascinating new discovery – and way more pleasing – was that a man can have an orgasm despite the fact that his penis is entirely flaccid. I was amazed and very pleased with this new knowledge. My new technique of 'licky-sucky' rehabilitation began.

There was considerable personal pain during these early days post-surgery. I found it extremely painful to see Alan's distress at having lost his precious 'cherry'. He had fought so hard, for so many years, to keep prostate cancer at bay. He viewed his current situation as a kind of personal failure.

Then there was concern at seeing Alan's penis in its new state; smaller, icy cold and bluey purple in colour. I couldn't help thinking that the circulation to his dick was not working very well at all. Again, my answer was – and still is – licky-sucky! It is my firm belief – not to be shaken by any hard scientific facts to the contrary, if there are any – that frequent, regular stimulation of the penis is crucial if you want to get any improvement.

I can't stress strongly enough how important it is for you and your partner to be as loving, patient and physically demonstrative as possible. Hugs, cuddles, kissing and verbal positivity are critical for both parties. I have met a few women who were not so supportive and it really made me sad.

As I write this chapter, it is approximately 18 months down the track from Alan's surgery. Sex these days is certainly different from how it was before the op. Viagra™

is not the magic bullet that we thought it might be, but it does help. It seems to me that, as time goes on, the little blue pills have an increasingly positive effect on Mr Percy. Again, plenty of stimulation and laughter really help.

The Trimix™ injection method is more predictable. Personally, I hate this technique. I really don't like seeing Alan go through the pain of the injection – usually it's when the solution enters the bloodstream that seems to cause the most discomfort and not the initial sting of the needle. The resulting stiffy is not like the ones we enjoyed pre-surgery. Generally, Trimix™ results in a fuller penis, but it's not as rigid as a true erection. We can and do have sex after Alan jabs himself, but I always fear the potential for scar tissue from the needle.

Any words of advice that I have for other partners of men with prostate cancer can be listed in point form:

- Be kind and patient.
- Communicate – listen to your partner and share your own feelings as well.
- Laugh as often as possible with your partner – especially when having or attempting sex.
- Show plenty of affection – physically and in other ways.
- Always be positive that things can and will improve for both of you.

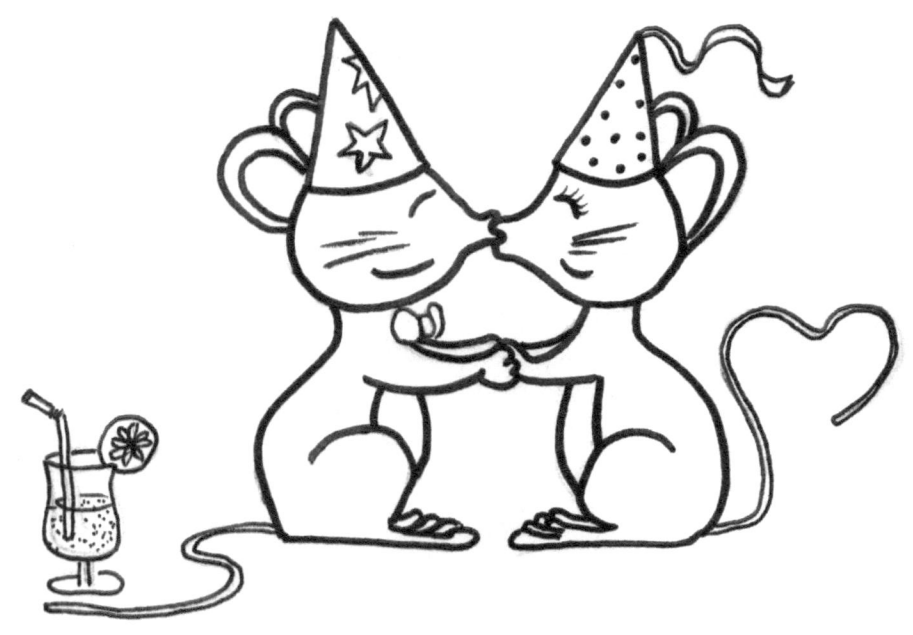

15. Be Kind to Yourself and Ask for Help

"How are you feeling?" This is a question I was asked whenever I was with friends or family. It was the tone of the question that I sensed to mean "are you alright? No cancer stuff?" I felt that there was genuine concern. Yes, I was feeling well, I was keeping fit, watched what I ate, everything in balance. I kept an eye on the stress in my life; like stepping down from some of the volunteer roles that I had been involved with over the past three years or so.

In fact, I realised that I went back too early to one organisation I was involved with; thus denying myself plenty of time to recover on all levels. In 2011, I felt that I should be looking for a job, which put undue pressure on me. Often I just didn't feel like doing anything, and then there were the emotional and physical aspects of the after-effects of the operation. I needed to come to terms with the changes that had occurred to me, and also to Fiona.

When I look back at 2011 and, in particular, around the middle of that year, I can see I was not in a good space, and there was anger that I was attempting to deal with in different ways. What was this anger about? Well, there were a number of issues, and some had probably been sitting there for a while. Some were to do with the whole operation and its aftermath, my inability to stay on top of the prostate problem, and missing out on jobs.

Even though I did go back for counselling, I should have gone earlier. So, for those men out there who are finding the journey a bit of a struggle, seek help. Whether it be talking to your partner, a friend, Lifeline, Men's Line or counselling; you need to get your head around what is going on for you, and come to grips with the changes that you are facing.

You don't have to do it the hard way on your own; seeking help is not a sign of weakness. It shows strength to acknowledge that all is not well. Not getting help will, in turn, have a ripple effect on all your relationships, personal and otherwise.

16. There is Light at the End of the Tunnel

Certainly, there have been numerous milestones that happened in the 18 months or so after the operation. Things like coming down in pad sizes. The ability to walk around at home without my jocks on first thing in the morning, without fear of leaking or dribbling. The relief of not going to the toilet every half hour or so, or having to look for the toilet when I'm out and about.

There was also the relief of reaching the point where I only had to wear a small number one pad inside my jocks, and then, better still, going without any pads at all, yeah!

Then there was the ability to actually have an orgasm, without an erection, so soon after the operation. Of overcoming the frustration – and working on relaxing – when attempting to have sex. Becoming aware and accepting that, over time, it may just take longer to reach an orgasm. This meant taking a different view and approach to having sex, and making better use of my imagination, and being persistent.

This is not bragging, it's to let men (and partners) know that it can happen; it may take a bit of perseverance but, in my experience, it can happen.

Do not give up, ever! Talk to your partner, communicate how you feel, keep close, cuddle, touch, experiment with what does and doesn't work for both of you.

Give all the tablets a go, even though they may take a while to kick in; one type may work better for you than another, but check with your GP first if you have any heart problems.

Towards the end of that first 18 months, there was a healing process occurring within, concerning the way the nerves down below receive messages from the brain. I call this 'the tingles' and it occurs when we play around, being frisky. It's as if there is an awakening going on down below, and this is even more apparent when I fantasise, which adds to the reaction from Percy, who seemed to be more responsive to the stimulation he received. There was more fullness happening. Of course, it was still nowhere near what Percy used to be, but changes were happening.

I continued to see Dr Dowker to keep everything on track and maintain my healing. I took the appropriate supplements to keep my system healthy, and ensured that I kept the fitness routine going, without overdoing it.

Since the operation, I found that, if I overdid things, there was a return of that deep tiredness I experienced immediately after the operation when working on some volunteer stuff. When I have really pushed myself, that tiredness returns.

I have also allowed myself time out more often, like walking to the beach and not rushing back to do some job. I have given myself permission to meet friends for coffee, or even take an afternoon nap. This meant listening to my body.

There are men out there who are still working. Take it easy as much as you can to allow your body to heal. We are not machines and, yes, you can push yourself and get back into it, but who says you have to? There's no medal for going back to work too early!

A number of studies have found that working on your fitness and exercising generally assists in reducing fatigue and aids recovery after an operation.

16. There is Light at the End of the Tunnel

I cannot recommend too strongly that, after your treatment, you give serious thought to seeing a health professional who is experienced in kinesiology, chiropractic, or osteopathy. I believe these treatments can be useful in the healing process.

A number of osteopaths also practise a therapy called 'craniosacral' or 'cranial-sacral'; this too can prove useful in bringing the body to a state of health and assisting with the healing process, on all levels. I am only speaking from my experience, but having treatments with Eric and the osteopaths has certainly made a difference to my health and wellbeing. I also had some acupuncture with a colleague, Dr David Wang, to help the healing along.

I also had some reflexology treatments on my feet, focusing on the bladder-urinary areas and related points. I believe that these treatments made some changes to my bladder and how it works, mostly increasing the length of time between visits to the toilet, and fewer feelings of needing to urinate. I felt that my bladder function was more 'normal'; there was the occasional leak, but I found I could stand for longer without the leaks happening as much.

Sexually, things were slowly improving, again possibly due to the treatments I was receiving, and the nerves themselves also healing. I even noticed some fullness in Percy in the mornings when I woke up to go the toilet – not that he had a full-on 'piss horn' like I would get prior to the operation, but hope springs eternal! I was still doing the injections to achieve a full erection. I had contemplated the vacuum pumps, but decided to go down that path only if I could no longer tolerate the injections.

17. Things to Consider If Diagnosed with Prostate Cancer

The following points are only my thoughts and experiences, having been down the prostate cancer track, and having thought a great deal about things after the event. Always bear in mind that every diagnosis will bring its unique treatment, depending on the individual's health and wellbeing.

Wherever possible, seek a second opinion and advice from another specialist. For example, in Melbourne, the Alfred Hospital has a Prostate Cancer Centre which offers all types of treatment and, given your diagnosis, can assist you in determining which treatment will best suit you and your situation.

As tempting as it is, use Google™ with caution. Use only reputable medical sites and beware of others offering cures of all sorts. By all means, look at what has worked for other men, and if you have decided on active surveillance, then work on your health and fitness. Complementary therapies may prove useful in assisting you in your journey of healing.

Your mental approach is also important, so look at what

will support you and your partner and, if that means getting counselling, then do that; develop a 'can do' approach to the situation. Remember, every man is different, as is each situation and diagnosis – we are all unique.

If there is a Prostate Cancer Support Group in your area, attending it may prove to be useful. Typically, you can hear how other men and their partners dealt with prostate cancer, as well as what types of treatments individuals within the group had used, and what they decided did and didn't work. Of course, there is the emotional support that comes from attending a group to share experiences. Some men just want to gather information and move on, and that is fine too. If the group doesn't work for you, that's okay.

Remember that each of us will differ in how we respond to treatment; even if you and I have the same treatment, we will have our own individual responses, recovery and journeys. Our journey will be subjective and will be based on our own sense of reality. We have our own filters through which we view life's events and react accordingly.

Treat this episode in your life as an investment, if you like, in that you will seek out all information, sorting the wheat from the chaff. Gather information, talk to your family/partner, seek the best option for you and what you feel comfortable with. Do not let others bully, intimidate or scare you into a treatment you are not sure of, or do not want.

An important part of this journey is to get all the facts about the after-effects of all the treatments, and how and what you can do to deal with them. Don't be put off by evasive answers.

I have often heard that men, when diagnosed with prostate cancer, will say to the specialist "What would you do in my position?" The answer may be insightful at the least! Remember, it is your body, your decision, along with input from your partner/family, and your medical specialist(s).

Diagnosis of prostate cancer can be major wake-up call for most men. If you are finding the journey a bit of a struggle, seek assistance. Talk to your partner and be honest about your feelings; that may mean crying, being angry and everything in between.

Discuss your fears, whether it be incontinence, lack of erections, or having to use a needle to get an erection, or even how you might view yourself differently as a man. Let your close friends know, so they can be a source of support and, if need be, seek counselling to keep yourself mentally strong.

Avoid sitting on your emotions and feelings, not dealing with them, otherwise they may pop up in the near future when you least expect them. So, go with the flow and let them out; they are part of who we are, as human and emotional beings – we are social animals – they are part of our psyche.

With over 25 years' experience working in natural therapies and 10 years' plus in counselling, I have had clients who experienced past memories, feelings and emotions that had not been dealt with. In particular, I have come across some men who, even two or three years after having treatment for prostate cancer, are still dealing with their emotions regarding the after-effects of the treatment – including not being given all the facts about that treatment by their specialist.

Whatever helps you get through this period and beyond, stick with it, but ensure it's a positive approach. We are mental, emotional, physical and spiritual beings, so be open to all experiences and a possible range of emotions and feelings that may surface. This time will certainly make you very aware of being alive – some say this event helped them re-evaluate their lives and what was important to them, like a tap on the shoulder.

When you do go to see the specialist(s), take a list of questions to ask and take your partner along for support – they may also have questions. I have heard of men taking a voice-recorder to the appointment, so they can review what was said, and what they may not have heard – you might be surprised at what you miss.

Don't forget your physical health. If you have time, work on your fitness prior to the operation or whatever treatment you decide on. Exercise is good for your physical and mental wellbeing, whether or not you have prostate cancer.

And if it's active surveillance that you choose, then your fitness is critical, along with your diet. And remain positive about your choice!

Finally, once you've decided on the most appropriate treatment, after taking into consideration the best advice and information available, then make that decision final. Close off the other options, and put all your energy into whatever you have to do to get through this time and beyond.

Focus on a positive outcome, take care of yourself on all levels, give yourself time to heal, depending on the treatment you have, and avoid rushing back into daily life – you may be affected more than you realise.

Once again, we are all different and will respond and heal differently, depending on what is going on in our lives at the time. I am still amazed at how some men bounce back so quickly, have little incontinence, are able to get their erections back fast, and – at least on the surface – appear 'together'. This just demonstrates the huge range in how individuals deal with adversity and the challenges in life.

If you, the reader, have only learned one new thing from this book, then it has been worthwhile. Of course, writing this book has been a personal journey for me from the outset. I needed to get my experiences and feelings onto paper, in the hope that, by telling how it was – good, bad, ugly and funny – other men may not feel so alone. If you, the reader, are facing an operation, this book may have helped you to know what to expect afterwards, including ways to deal with incontinence, the sex stuff, and everything else.

I am not aware of any magic diet, exercise or other 'thing' that will prevent prostate cancer. I know there are books out there that claim all sorts of things, so if you do read them, look for other evidence, and remember that we all respond differently to supplements.

Of course, things may change in the near future. Certainly,

having a healthy diet, regular exercise, and balance in your life may go some way towards reducing the chances, but life is full of changes and challenges. Genetics is another possible contributor to the mix; there is a statistically higher chance of being diagnosed with prostate cancer if you have a family history on either parent's side. And if there is family history of prostate cancer, all the more reason to take care of your health.

Having said that, I noticed in my past pathology reports that my vitamin D levels were low, so I started taking a vitamin D capsule. Research has shown a possible link between low vitamin D levels in men and prostate cancer. There is some difference of opinions about what constitutes 'low', but generally anything below 50 nmol/L would need to be looked at.

In my case, in May 2010, the vitamin D level was 101 nmol/L. In December 2010, it had dropped to 57, possibly because I had not been consistent in taking the supplement. It was in December 2010 that I had the DRE and the prostate was found to be firm! So was there some connection? Possibly so, but I will never know. Considering that most of the general population is supposed to be vitamin D deficient, you might wish to ask your doctor to add the vitamin D test to your usual annual blood testing procedures (e.g. cholesterol, glucose and PSA).

Also, get the test done early in the week, as I have read that vitamin D levels in the blood sample can drop off after it is taken, and the longer it takes for the pathology lab to do the tests, the more likely the level of vitamin D will decline. Of course, having a healthy vitamin D level is also good for your general health and wellbeing.

The important thing to remember is to have regular health check-ups with your doctor, developing a relationship with him/her, so that you feel comfortable talking to them about all health matters. When you reach 40, if there is a family history of prostate cancer, make sure to include the PSA blood test, as well as a free-to-total PSA, as part of your annual pathology check-up. The free-to-total PSA levels will give you additional information – potentially critical information – about how your prostate is functioning.

I am happy to hear readers' thoughts about this book, and whether it has been useful or not. Remember to pass it on to others to read, so more people can be informed and aware of what to expect. Thank you for taking the time to read about my prostate adventures – I hope they will be useful for your own life's journey.

Postscript: Two Years On

As the anniversary of the removal of my prostate came around, and I was tidying up this story, I realised that there have been further changes on a number of levels for me. I thought it might be useful to include these changes, to finish on a positive note.

Remember, every man is different and will heal and respond in their own way depending on the treatment they receive.

The following comments are not in any particular order, but represent more of the sign-posts along the way as changes were occurring for me.

Going back to counselling at the Veterans' Counselling Service, I realised that I was still struggling with my self-image insofar as being able to have sex and all that having sex entailed. Even though we went over previous stuff that had been discussed in the sessions, it was helpful to review what was still running around in my head.

I also realised that only I can make the changes and determine how I think and operate in a different way; not so much a new me, but a transition to a different way of functioning.

I also continued to experience the niggling in the back of my mind about my decision to have the prostate removed. It was during these counselling sessions that the emotions rose up again, a mixture of - Did I do the right thing? – Why didn't I stop and step back to give alternatives another go? – What was really going on at the time? - and a sense of not being in control.

I had to keep reminding myself that the prostate biopsy showed aggressive cells present, so alternatives were not an option. Soon it became clear to me that going around in these circles was not helpful at all, on a number of levels. So, with the counsellor's assistance, three positive statements were drafted that I would look at every time I started to re-hash all that stuff from the past.

There were positive things happening; once I finished the reflexology sessions, I continued to rub those points on my feet and face that related to the bladder and related areas. I felt that there had been a marked improvement in my incontinence. I was going longer between toilet visits and managed some nights not getting up at all, which meant a full night's sleep – wonderful.

There was the occasional slip-up, like bending over or lifting up an object, and not pulling up on the pelvic floor muscles first. Because there was some urine sitting in the urethra, out it would pop, a run of urine, sometimes just a drop or two, other times more than that. Well, enough to leave a reasonable wet spot in the jocks. I found that annoying, but overall the time between visits to the toilet has become longer, up to three hours at a time. I learned to resist going to the toilet 'just in case', by doing the quick pelvic floor clench to reduce the urge of wanting to go.

I found myself mentally and emotionally in a better space. There were the occasional days when I felt I was starting to revisit the past and that was not helpful, so I took action to get out of that space. These feelings could be triggered by a TV show or by something I was reading.

I had been involved for some time in delivering talks on prostate cancer on behalf of the Prostate Cancer Foundation, which included having available various publications from the Foundation and BeyondBlue. I realised, on reflection, that I could have been better informed, and even read some of the publications from these two organisations. Even though I was reasonably aware of what to expect, the consequences, and after-effects of the operation, it would have been useful if I had read more so that I was a bit more prepared for the possible reactions emotionally, at least for myself and Fiona.

That is just hindsight, which is of no use to me now, except to encourage other men and their partners to avail themselves of the various publications so they may be informed of what to expect if they are facing treatment for prostate cancer, or any other cancer.

I realised that talking to Fiona about what I was thinking helped to get these thoughts out of my head and focused more on the future. Ruminating about what I could have or should have done in the past was not helpful to me in any way.

As for the sexual aspect and the after-effects, there continues to be ongoing improvement. I am still injecting myself to get a full erection, and lately find that my erections feel firmer, a bit like they used to be. Of course, it does take a bit longer to feel as if there is any sensation happening – not that Fiona is complaining – and it does take longer to reach a climax, depending on how often we have been intimate. But, boy, when it does happen, it's pretty mind-blowing, minus the ejaculation of course. There is an occasional slightly painful feeling to the orgasms, but these are also becoming less frequent over time and that is influenced by a number of different issues.

I am still using the blue pill from time to time, but that means taking it on an empty stomach, so a bit more planning is involved. Percy's reaction to it does not result in a full erection, so a lot of stimulation or fantasy is required. Again, perseverance and willingness to attempt different approaches all help to get you towards whatever works for both of you.

I know the nerves surrounding the prostate that were

affected by the operation are coming back to life, due to the fact that Percy responds a lot more when I fantasise. A partial erection occurs, not a full-on erection, but at least something happens, and then we take it from there. Another sign that the nerves are working is that I often wake up in the morning with a partial erection when going to the toilet. Again, it's not the full-on one I used to get before the operation, but it does happen, so hope springs eternal!

Each couple, of course, will deal with the sexual or intimacy issue differently, depending on their age, general health, and how sexually active they were before the treatment. If you are both willing to continue with that part of your relationship, then do so. Seek information, read what others have done, but the important thing to remember is that all couples are different and need to discover what gives them the most pleasure when being intimate and sexual. You may just have to find an alternative path from what you did before.

As I reviewed the last few years, I saw that it has been a journey of changes, learning, adapting and being flexible, which is most important. In fact, we don't have that much control at times over our lives, which can be most frustrating and stressful. It often means living one day at a time and enjoying the moment, whatever you are doing.

What you do have control over, to some degree, is your health and that involves the choices you make daily about what you eat, drink, think and feel, being physically active, and how you react to others and society at large. I believe these can all impact on our health.

Postscript: Five Years On

As I started to make some decisions about publishing, I realised that I was reaching the five year survival mark, and statistics state that 95% of men after the operation will be alive; of course men can die from other causes. And after 10 years around 85% of men are still alive.

There are similar figures for those men who decide on doing active surveillance, in that after 10 years the survival rate is similar to men having the operation.

Not that I am dwelling on this fact, but getting to the five year mark, with overall good health is a positive point. It is a good reminder to keep focusing on my health and wellbeing, and ensure that I keep doing whatever is necessary to stay healthy and not contribute to the cancer coming back.

My PSA levels since the operation had remained at 0.05 from March 2011 till May 2013, and then from December 2013 dropped to 0.01 and stayed there, which means the PSA is barely detectable.

Unfortunately for some men, this is not the case. Even though they may be given the all clear after their operation, somehow the prostate cancer has gone walk about and their PSA is on the rise, so that they may now be looking at hormonal treatments or radiation therapy.

For this to happen is devastating for them and their family, so I can only think I have been lucky to have caught mine early enough, before it had gone walk-about.

Your overall health is directly affected by what you eat and drink, your emotional and mental state, and how active you are; so take every opportunity to stay healthy. We don't know how long we have on this planet, and remember, **this is not a dress rehearsal**.

So at this point in time – 2016 – there have been a number of improvements and, looking back, I can now see what I was experiencing, and hopefully provide some positive comments for you if facing a similar situation.

Waterworks!

The incontinence is good, although if I am to be out and standing for some time I still put in the number one pad, just in case. I am certainly aware of keeping the water up and not going to the toilet unless I have to. I can hold on for a couple of hours or so, which is great.

But there are the intermittent leaks from time to time, like when I kneel down and even though I have been to the toilet, there is a little leak – a bit annoying. Or, for some reason, I seem to have to go to the toilet more often than usual, but that is the exception rather than the rule and certainly not the norm.

When I compare myself to how some other men are experiencing incontinence, I am okay; I keep doing the pelvic floor exercises and engage in regular physical activity.

And yes, I still sit to take a leak generally at home, and certainly when I get up in the middle of the night. Of course I am also 'milking the urethra' to encourage the emptying of any urine that may still be sitting in the urethra after having a leak, and I give Percy a good shake to make sure that it is all gone.

Sometimes, I will wake up in the early hours of the morning and wonder if I need to go again. Does the bladder need emptying again, or is it the urethra sending the signal? So I do the quick clenches – pulling the pelvic floor muscles about six times – sometimes that does the trick and I can go back to sleep.

Occasionally that doesn't work, so I get up for another leak. What doesn't help is drinking any liquids too late at night, meaning that I will be more likely to have to get up for a pee.

Anything else that happens in this area is very much an individual's experience, due to any number of circumstances relating to their general health before and after surgery; doing pelvic floor exercises, how each person's body heals, and what they do to assist the body in that area.

Medical Advances

Every year new medical treatments are being developed, with greater involvement of medical technology and the whole biomedical field. Recently, there has been the development of a new MRI scanning procedure which takes an image of the prostate to obtain a better view of where the prostate cancer cells are growing within the gland.

Other recent treatment advances include the Nano knife, an ultra-high-frequency ultrasound. There is also the development of high-voltage electricity to treat the prostate, which appears to be having some success.

However, as in all cases to do with prostate cancer, each treatment and its success or otherwise will depend on your health, age, other health problems, the stage of the cancer and whether you are actually a candidate for the treatment, along with the experience of the treating surgeon.

In some respects, by contacting a local prostate cancer support group, you might learn about other possible treatment options. This may save you some time in attempting to find out what medical treatments are on offer. It is always best to discuss possible treatment approaches with your GP or specialist medical advisor. Remember, what works for one man does not necessarily work for all.

The Sex Stuff

Well, this has improved in different ways. Again, I have to say that every man will recover from their operation differently and heal differently. Your age at the time of the operation, how sexually active you have been, and pre-operative preparation will also influence how well you recover your erections. Another vital factor is how much your partner is involved in this sexual healing aspect.

So am I getting erections like I used to? No, I am not; but the fantasising is having results in that I do get half an erection and Percy now reacts fairly quickly to the scenes in my mind. I also get what I call the tingles down deep in the lower abdomen when this occurs, which to me at least means the nerves are responding.

You may find that with lots of physical touching, caressing and even massage, Percy will start to become erect and ready for whatever follows. Not that having a massage has to lead to sex!

I am no longer taking the little blue pill or others, but I continue to use Trimix™ injections. Even though I would rather not have to, at the moment it is a fact of life that if I/we want to have sex then I have to inject myself.

We (Fiona and I) have attempted other ways – foreplay, etc. where I start off with half an erection, albeit a bit soft, and then I might be able to enter Fiona and the erection does in part become harder, but for some reason it does not stay that way. Again, this depends on the circumstances at the time. As one of the men at the local support group said "sometimes it's like trying to play snooker with a piece of rope"!

Also, during these moments the sensitivity feels a lot less, so that seems to add to loss of the erection. But then there are other times when it all works out, so there is no consistent pattern as to what works and does not. Of course, oral sex never fails to get an erection (unless I am very tired and trying too hard) and the subsequent orgasm is amazing, but different each time.

On the other hand, using the Trimix™ injections and

subsequent erection that occurs certainly allows us to be fully intimate. When I do enter Fiona, the erection becomes even harder and the sensitivity feels more normal, although that can depend on the position, and how long it has been since we last had sex.

The orgasms continue to be amazing, without the ejaculation of course, although sometimes the sensation during an orgasm somehow feels like I am ejaculating.

I have also found with the Trimix™, which has an expiry date on the bottle, that the longer I go past the use by date, the more Trimix™ I have to draw up into the injection vial to get a decent erection. If the Trimix™ is fresh, then I can get away with only using around 80cc of the fluid.

Apart from the initial sting of the needle going into Percy, I find that there is a real sting from the fluid once it is fully injected, but this lasts only for a few seconds.

Another member of the local prostate support group told me that he found, by slowly wriggling the needle as he injected himself, the needle seemed to go in a bit easier. So I now do that – slowly of course – and it seems to help. I also found that by injecting the solution as I pushed the needle into Percy, the needle in turn was able to go further into Percy.

The important thing is that you and your partner continue to be sexually intimate, in whatever way works for both of you. As for the sex act, if penetration is not your thing, then finding other ways to be close and intimate, where you both feel satisfied and desirable, is part of the healing process.

The act of waking up with some resemblance of an erection in the morning has certainly changed; from a sort of half-soft erection to not much at all. Remember that, prior to an operation to remove the prostate, most men would wake up with an erection in the morning as part of the body's process of supplying fresh blood and oxygen to their penis.

As I have said earlier in the book, a man has got to keep the blood and oxygen flowing into his penis to keep it healthy after the operation. You can do that by being sexual, masturbating, injecting, using the little blue pill, or the vacuum device to get blood into Percy. It's another one of those changes that you have to deal with after the operation.

With both of us now working, finding or making the time to be intimate, along with me having to inject myself first, it can at times take the shine off the whole thing. But a man's got to do what a man's got to do, and that is keep the wife happy!

All jokes aside, we certainly enjoy the moment of sexual intimacy, and when it's been a while, that intimacy is even better, what else can I say! And there is the laying in bed together afterwards, enjoying that post-orgasm euphoria sleep.

And Life Goes On

Another milestone that occurred for me was making the decision to go back to work as a Counsellor and Natural Health Practitioner. I found a health centre that was expanding in Black Rock, and after speaking with Marta, the Naturopath, was able to join her team.

I am working two to three days a week and feeling a lot happier being back in that role as I gain a lot of satisfaction from my work. I now feel that I have a purpose in life that is fulfilling; in particular, counselling men who are also facing a prostate cancer diagnosis, and having to make decisions around treatments and their side-effects, emotionally and physically.

When I look back over the last five years, I realise that I probably was struggling at times with what had occurred, and of course I had gone back to receive counselling to get over that hurdle.

More recently, on re-reading information about depression and anxiety, I think I may have been experiencing this to some degree, but I put that down to pressuring myself too much to get back into the workforce and, to some extent, on expecting my body to heal ASAP.

About two years after my operation, my wife Fiona, was found to have cancer of the stomach lining. So she changed her diet, took specific supplements, and the next scan did not show any cancer. Fantastic!

But, the radiation oncologist suggested that just because it was not detectable didn't mean it wasn't there, bummer!

After some discussion, Fiona decided to have the radiotherapy, which was another bit of stress to face, for both of us; I believe it probably contributed to the fact that I was not travelling too well. Of course Fiona had to deal with three weeks of radiotherapy and subsequent side-effects in the following months.

After Fiona's radiotherapy sessions were done with, I went back to see a counsellor to address the issues I had been dealing with. The good news is that Fiona got over that ordeal and is now back at work and well. Nothing like a few hurdles to jump over to see how we deal with the challenges that pop up.

Now what? Often it is one day at a time, so that keeps the stress to a manageable level; not thinking too far ahead, as that can lead to anxiety about what you can and cannot do about different situations. Avoid revisiting the past, worrying over what you should, might, or could have done. That only adds to thinking that you didn't make the right decision.

A while ago at a counselling session, the counsellor came up with the following statements for me to refer to when I found myself revisiting my decision:

> My health reflects that I made the right choice.
>
> I made the right choice with the information I had at the time.
>
> I did make the right choice.

Of course, the above statements in some cases for men may mean SFA (SWEET F*** ALL), as they may feel they were pushed, rushed or not given enough information at the time of diagnosis. I have come across men who have felt this and it is a difficult one for them to come to terms with, and it can impact on them in different ways.

My only suggestion in this situation is that if you are still struggling with past events, it may be worth considering some counselling to assist in getting you to a better place mentally and emotionally. Your quality of life is also affected by what you are thinking.

With all major decisions in life, we attempt to get all relevant information before moving forward. In relation to a prostate cancer diagnosis, getting all the facts is important, and considering the side-effects from each of the treatment options. More importantly though, ask yourself whether you can live with the particular side-effects from the decision you are about to make.

This is where it might be worthwhile involving your partner, family, close friend or carer; talking through, with them, the options that you are considering. You could also see a counsellor to work through the issues you are facing, as this may go some way towards becoming clearer about the decision process that you are undertaking.

If you are not faced with such a decision and you are reading this book out of curiosity perhaps, or to know about what a man may face after an operation, then I hope this book proves worthwhile.

And Finally, Taking Care of Yourself

I encourage all men to take charge of their health and wellbeing, and to have regular twelve-monthly health check-ups, like you would service your car. Your body will keep running without check-ups, but something, somewhere in your body may start to run rough! And then it will take a lot more effort, time, energy and money to get back on track.

In fact, it comes down to this - who's going to take care of you if you don't? How well do you take care of yourself? Do you need to make some improvements in this area?

Final Word from Fiona – Five Years On

Alan is still alive. That's the most important thing as far as I'm concerned.

Prostate cancer can kill and yet it rarely captures the public imagination (or publicity) as breast cancer does. Like breast cancer, prostate cancer strikes at the core of a person's sexual identity. I've watched Alan's suffering and I've also seen other men who have struggled with the disease and with the outcomes of their individual treatment decisions.

My message to people reading this book is that love and support are absolutely vital ingredients for a true recovery from prostate cancer and its various forms of treatment. If you are in a relationship, make sure that you give one another as much care and affection as possible, and never stop communicating. Be courageous and share your fears, your anger, your sadness and your yearnings.

Since Alan had his prostate removed, I can honestly say that I think we have become closer and understand one another better. Our sex life is very different now from what it was prior to the operation. But different is okay. We may have lost spontaneity, but we still have loads of fun. Penetration does feel different (usually not as intense), but it does feel good.

Can I honestly say that sex is as good as it used to be pre-op? No. There are times when Alan uses the Trimix™ and "sticks himself", but his dick just doesn't get hard enough. Oral sex, though, works every time!

Spooning in bed after sex (no matter how successful) is always wonderful – it seems to bring us closer and certainly makes me feel particularly happy. I remain a dedicated "pouncer" and have a tendency to touch Alan a lot. I am so proud of him and so glad to have him in my life.

Dealing with Alan's emotions over the past five years has sometimes been difficult. He does go through times when he tends to dwell on his decision to have surgery. He gets particularly agitated about it when he learns about new treatment possibilities – I suppose that is understandable.

Alan has poured so much of his energy into helping other men deal with their prostate cancer diagnoses. He has delivered talks and presentations, facilitated the local Prostate Cancer Support Group, helped raise awareness about the disease and conducted fundraising to aid research. I am so proud of his efforts.

Over the past five years, I have observed many men joke about prostate cancer – the "old man's disease". I am sick and tired of the silly jokes about digital rectal examination. Men have a responsibility, not just to themselves, but to all their family, friends, work colleagues and, especially, their partners, to take this subject seriously. Too many men dismiss the idea of getting tested. Too many men bury their heads in the sand.

I feel passionately that men need to "man up" and take responsibility for their own health. I say, don't wait for your GP to raise the subject – some never will. Be persistent and make sure that you seek out the information you need to know about this disease – it doesn't only strike old men and when it happens to younger men it is often more aggressive.

We live in a culture that is saturated in sex, but afraid

to talk about it in an open, honest and down-to-earth way. Australians are so fond of using humour to deflect subjects that they don't want to face – I say that it's time to grow up and develop some emotional intelligence. Women die from breast cancer and men die from prostate cancer. They can also survive, and their lives post-treatment can be wonderful and fulfilling. That's what I would definitely prefer.

References

Arndt, Bettina. *What men want in Bed*. 2010. Melbourne University Press, Victoria, Australia.

Doidge, Norman, M.D. *The brain that changes itself — Stories of personal triumph from the frontiers of brain science*. 2008. Scribe Publications, Victoria, Australia.

Dornan, Peter. *Conquering incontinence — A new and physical approach to a freer lifestyle*. 2003. Allen & Unwin, New South Wales, Australia.

Rashid, Prem, Associate Professor. *Prostate Cancer — Your guide to the disease, treatment options and outcomes*. 3rd ed. 2010. Uronorth Group, New South Wales, Australia.

Resources

The following list is certainly not exhaustive, but should give readers a helpful starting point.

Books
Alschuler, Lisa N, ND, FABNO, and Gazella, Karolyn A. *The Definitive Guide to Thriving After Cancer: A Five-Step Integrative Plan to Reduce the Risk of Recurrence and Build Lifelong Health.* 2011. Ten Speed Press, Berkeley, USA.

Arndt, Bettina. *What Men Want in Bed.* 2010. Melbourne University Press, Victoria, Australia.

Bays, Brandon. *The Journey™.* 1999. Harper Element, Hammersmith, London, UK.

Béliveau, Richard, PhD and Gingras, Denis, PhD. *Foods that Fight Cancer — Preventing and Treating Cancer through Diet.* 2006. Allen & Unwin, Crows Nest, New South Wales, Australia.

Chambers, Suzanne, Professor. *Facing the Tiger. A Guide for Men with Prostate Cancer and the People Who Love Them.* 2013. Australian Academic Press Group Pty Ltd, Toowong, Queensland, Australia.

Doidge, Norman, M.D. *The brain that changes itself — Stories of personal triumph from the frontiers of brain science.* 2008. Scribe Publications, Victoria, Australia.

Doran, Peter. *Conquering Incontinence. A new and physical approach to a freer lifestyle.* 2013. Allen & Unwin, Crows Nest, New South Wales, Australia.

Hay, Louise L. *You can heal your life.* 1988. Specialist Publications, Concord, New South Wales, Australia.

Lawrenson, Alan G. *An ABC of Prostate Cancer in 2015.* 2014. Self-published, Pretty Beach, New South Wales, Australia (to be reprinted as *ABC of Prostate Cancer treatments*).

Myers, Charles "Snuffy", Dr. *Beating Prostate Cancer: Hormonal Therapy and Diet.* 2007. Rivanna Health Publications, Earlysville, Virginia, USA.

Ortner, Nick. *The Tapping Solution — A revolutionary system for stress-free living.* 2013. Hay House, California, USA.

Rashid, Prem, Associate Professor. *Prostate Cancer — Your guide to the disease, treatment options and outcomes.* 3rd ed. 2010. Uronorth Group, New South Wales, Australia.

Servan-Schreiber, David, Dr. Anti Cancer — *A new way of life.* 2008. Scribe, Brunswick, Victoria, Australia.

Websites and Organisations Within Australia

Alfred Hospital's Melbourne Prostate Institute
www.melbourneprostate.org

Andrology Australia
www.andrologyaustralia.org

Australian Advanced Prostate Cancer Support Groups
www.jimjimjimjim.com

Australian Centre for Prostate Cancer and Men's Health
www.prostatecancerresearch.org.au

Australian Commonwealth Department of Health site for palliative care
www.health.gov.au/palliativecare

Banksia Palliative Care
www.banksiapalliative.com.au

Beyondblue
www.beyondblue.org.au (Helpline 1300 22 4636)

Cancer Council Victoria
www.cancervic.org.au (Helpline 13 11 20)

Continence Foundation of Australia
www.continence.org.au (Helpline 1800 33 00 66)

Men's Helpline Australia
www.mensline.org.au (1300 789 978)

PFLEX Pty Ltd (pelvic floor exercise information and products for men and women)
www.pelvicfloorexercise.com.au (1300 763 940)

Prostate Cancer Foundation of Australia
www.pcfa.org.au

Prostmate
www.prostmate.org.au

The SA Prostate Cancer Clinical Outcomes Collaborative (SAPCOCC) (previously Lions Australia)
www.prostatehealth.org.au

Veterans and Veterans Families Counselling Service
www.vvcs.gov.au (1800 011 046)

Websites and Organisations Outside Australia

American Institute for Diseases of the Prostate (US)
www.prostateteam.com (Dr Charles "Snuffy" Myers)

Life Extension (US)
www.lef.org

National Cancer Institute (US)
www.cancer.gov

Prostate Cancer You're the Man (UK)
www.yourtheman.org

Scientific American
www.scientificamerican.com

Us TOO International Prostate Cancer Education and Support Network (US)
www.ustoo.org

USA Prostate Cancer Foundation
www.pcf.org

Notes

Notes

Notes

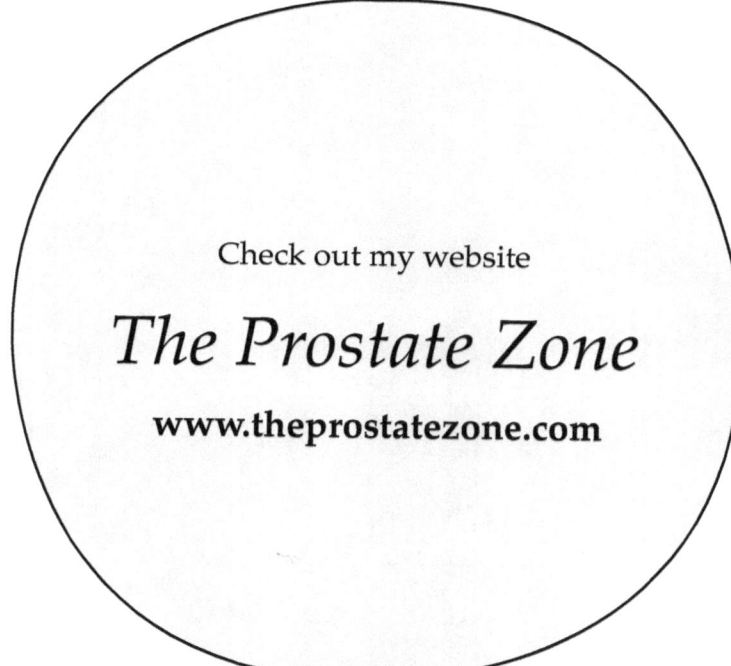

www.ingramcontent.com/pod-product-compliance
Lightning Source LLC
Chambersburg PA
CBHW021129300426
44113CB00006B/350